Mindful Medicine

40 SIMPLE PRACTICES TO HELP HEALTHCARE
PROFESSIONALS HEAL BURNOUT AND
RECONNECT TO PURPOSE

Jan Chozen Bays, MD

Author of *Mindfulness on the Go*

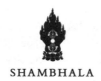

SHAMBHALA

Shambhala Publications, Inc.
2129 13th Street
Boulder, Colorado 80302
www.shambhala.com

Cover art: Lightspring / Shutterstock.com
Cover & interior design: Kate E. White

9 8 7 6 5 4 3 2 1

First Edition
Printed in the United States of America

Shambhala Publications makes every effort to print on acid-free, recycled paper.
Shambhala Publications is distributed worldwide by
Penguin Random House, Inc., and its subsidiaries.

LIBRARY OF CONGRESS CATALOGING-IN-PUBLICATION DATA
Names: Bays, Jan Chozen, author.
Title: Mindful medicine: 40 simple practices to help healthcare professionals heal burnout and reconnect to purpose / Jan Chozen Bays, MD.
Description: First edition. | Boulder, Colorado: Shambhala, [2022]
Identifiers: LCCN 2021056872 | ISBN 9781645470526 (trade paperback)
Subjects: LCSH: Mindfulness (Psychology) | Stress management. | Resilience (Personality trait)
Classification: LCC BF637.M56 B39 2022 | DDC 158.1/3—dc23/eng/20211217
LC record available at https://lccn.loc.gov/2021056872

This book is dedicated to those who willingly enter the trenches of human suffering, impelled by a fundamental vow to help relieve the pain and distress of others. May it inspire, support, and refresh you as you do this most important work.

Contents

Introduction

I am a pediatrician. I've worked at Kaiser Permanente and was on the faculty at a medical school. For thirty years, I worked in the field of child abuse at a hospital-based center in Oregon where we evaluated over one hundred cases of alleged abuse each month.

I know about physician burnout. From the inside. I know about compassion fatigue and secondary trauma. From the inside. I suddenly fell into these distressing states of heart and mind despite my forty-five years of sustained Zen meditation practice and despite all the markings of a successful career. I had published articles in medical journals and Buddhist magazines, lectured at international conferences on child abuse, learned acupuncture, established one of the first integrative medicine clinics in the United States, and taught meditation for decades. I had a happy marriage and family life and a lifelong, cheerful, and curious approach to everything I encountered.

How did this happen? When I had been doing child abuse work full-time for ten years, my father suddenly died of a stroke, and soon after, my Zen teacher also died. It is common for healthcare professionals to be able to maintain a demanding work schedule, coping well with frequent medical emergencies and tragedies—until something falls apart in their personal lives. One Friday night, after a week of particularly horrible child abuse cases, I was driving home two hours late because of a last-minute emergency rape exam on a teenager. A soppy country song began on the radio, and I found myself crying and afraid I would not be able to stop.

Over the next few weeks, I lost my appetite and began coming in to work late—just five or ten minutes—but late. I noticed that I was reactive, irritated with the coworkers who were my best friends. A call would come in from detectives at 5:15 p.m., asking if they could bring in an emergency case, and I found myself making any excuse not to see the child and to send them to the emergency room instead. When our evaluations helped authorities remove children from abusive homes, I saw some kids return to our program after suffering worse abuse in their foster home than in their family home. I began to wonder if our work was truly helpful or not.

I needed to understand what was happening to me; I needed a diagnosis, so I began to read. I discovered that I had all the symptoms of burnout: physical and emotional exhaustion, depression, depersonalization, and doubt in personal efficacy.[1] Burnout can happen to anyone in any profession, but it is particularly common among healthcare workers, emergency responders, and mental health and addiction specialists. When I realized the nature of my trouble, I also realized that I was likely the most resilient, equanimous person in the child abuse center where I was the medical director. If I was struggling emotionally and physically, I needed to learn about what was happening to me, the nature of my illness, and the treatment so that I could help myself and support my colleagues. Over the past twenty years, I have studied and lectured on burnout and developed mindfulness practices for people who work in the caring professions that can provide sustained well-being.

This little book is about what I learned. I hope it will be helpful for you.

The healthcare professions are in trouble. We lose more than one physician and nurse a day to suicide in the United States, the equivalent of two to three graduating classes of doctors and nurses each year. Among male physicians, suicide rates are 2–3 times the national average. Among female physicians, the completion rate of suicides is 2.5 to 4 times the general population.[2] Seventy percent of doctors do not recommend their profession to others, including—or especially—their children.[3]

First responders, including emergency medical technicians, firefighters, and police officers, also have higher suicide rates than average. More firefighters and police officers die by suicide than in the line of duty. A report on this phenomenon states, "Suicide is a result of mental illness, including depression and PTSD, which stems from constant exposure to death and destruction."[4]

I call this "working in the trenches of human suffering," experiencing things that other people do not ever want to experience or even hear us talk about. As I write, the COVID-19 pandemic has only worsened this situation.

During that week when we had three horrendous cases in a row at our child abuse center, our entire staff was traumatized, stunned, and grief-stricken. We asked our hospital chaplain for help. She explained that in the course of an ordinary human life (in a peace-time, developed country), people typically experience one traumatic event, such as the death of a parent, and have time to process and recover their emotional balance over the course of about a year. In contrast, many medical professionals and first responders often witness highly distressing events and have no time to recover before they move on to the next case or disaster. The chaplain called it "chronic acute stress" and compared it to soldiers in wartime who must "stuff" their grief and horror and continue fighting. She advised that protecting ourselves against the effects of these events requires unusual methods and spiritual support.

The unusual methods and spiritual support I and other healthcare workers have found to be most effective are an armamentarium of mindfulness practices and a regular meditation practice. I hope they will be equally effective for you.

There are various theories about why the joy drains out of medicine for so many of us: graduating with student loan debt that can take decades to work off; "assembly line" medicine with constant increases in paperwork and administrative burdens, leaving no time for true connection with patients; long, inflexible work hours plus on-call hours, adding up to little time for your family or yourself; the challenges of dealing with insurance companies and bureaucracies that seem uninterested in the plight of your patients; frustration with electronic medical records; and the stigma of admitting that you, who worked so hard for so many years to get where you are, are unhappy.

There are some (seemingly) simple solutions: Reduce your work hours. Hire someone to relieve you of administrative work. Find a practice situation that has more flexible hours. Say no kindly, but firmly.

When I was in the middle of burnout, my husband gave me a JUST SAY NO button to wear to work. Each evening, he'd ask how many times I had said no to someone's request for me to assume more responsibility. The answer was always a sheepish, "Zero." There is a catch-22 in medicine: If you refuse to do extra call, you are failing your patients and putting an extra burden on your coworkers. If you take a weekend off, you feel guilty about your friends who are still working. Next, he gave me a small metal clicker, the kind used by people with addictions to count the times the urge arises to use a substance. I still came home each night with zero on the clicker.

That's when I began to realize that I had a problem. I vowed to change. I remember how difficult it was the first time I said no. I got a call from a child abuse colleague, asking me to be the keynote speaker at a conference. I politely declined and said I could recommend someone else. They were disappointed, but I was firm, and trembling when I got off the phone. It was a beginning. I resigned after ten years of being the medical director and stepped back to be a child abuse examiner—a position with no administrative responsibilities and more connected to working with children—the work that drew me into the profession when I started. Eventually, I dropped to half-time, which actually meant working three-quarters time for half-pay, but I was happier. I was fortunate to be able to make this shift; not everyone with student loan debt and family obligations can do this. I started making clay sculptures and took square dancing lessons with my husband.

These changes were helpful, but there was still, deep inside like a buried splinter, something not quite right. I liked being a doctor and enjoyed my new free time activities, but I felt a lingering dissatisfaction. I needed a remedy that would work anytime, a door I could walk through anytime, anywhere, a door that would lead me to that place of simple presence that transforms irritation into curiosity, depression into equanimity, and clock-watching into the satisfying experience of flow.[5]

From my longtime Zen practice, I knew that meditation could open my mind to those positive states and help prepare me for an often-hectic day. But I needed ways to be able to open that door in the moment, when I wasn't on my meditation cushion, in the time between closing one exam room door and opening the next, while I listened to an angry patient or relative, as I washed my hands, as I sat my tired body down for a few blessed minutes to eat a few bites of lunch, or while I ran-walked to a conference or a code. I also needed ways to prepare my heart and mind for the coming day of encounters with the unknown, pleasant and not. I needed ways to clear out the day as it ended so I could be fully present with my husband and children.

In response to those challenges that every healthcare professional and emergency responder knows, I developed a number of mindfulness practices, guided meditations, and what I call "Rescue Remedies" for times of urgent need. These practices are similar to what I've shared in my previous books, like *Mindfulness on the Go*, but they are specifically tailored to the experiences, challenges, and gifts of people who work in healthcare in any way. I use these practices myself, and have found that they offered what I needed—ways to be with the inevitable challenges of healthcare work with more grace, self-compassion, and connection; ways to be present at work so I can be present out of work as well; and ways to reconnect to the passion that originally led me into the medical field.

I have shared these practices in a group called Mindful Medicine PDX—a weekly gathering of physicians, nurses, and other healthcare workers dedicated to sustaining and enhancing their work through mindfulness. We have also gathered for weekend retreats, where we practice and share in community in more depth. We have tried these practices and shaped them through our discoveries. They were particularly poignant during the COVID-19 crisis. I hope they will be as helpful to you as they have been to us.

HOW TO USE THIS BOOK

Mindful Medicine is for any person working on the front lines of human suffering. This includes doctors, nurses, nurse practitioners, certified nurse assistants, physician assistants, emergency medical technicians, and other first responders. I have the most experience working with people in healthcare settings, but I also write with the hope that many parts of this book might help support therapists of all kinds—physically and emotionally. Dentists and veterinarians have come to our weekly meetings and retreats, needing respite from their weariness and grief over all they've seen. We are so busy taking care of other people's children, parents, grandparents, or pets that we don't have time to take good care of ourselves. We see things that people outside our professions don't want to hear us talk about, and we don't usually have time to talk with each other except about the busyness at hand.

When there's an emergency, we can't stop to assess how the situation affects us. We can't arrive at a bad car wreck and spend time wailing about the unnecessary loss of life or being angry about people who drive drunk. We can't spend time weeping after an unsuccessful code on a young mother who had a cast put on her broken leg, stood up on her new crutches to leave with her family, and collapsed from a pulmonary embolus. We can't spend more than a few minutes telling a mother and father, called out of church to the hospital, that their son died of a gunshot wound in a botched robbery of a convenience store. We don't have time to grieve after a phone call informing us that a client has died by suicide; the next client is already in the waiting room.

We have to learn how to take care of ourselves in the moments that occur in our everyday life—as we commute to work, run to the ER, wait in the cafeteria line, or in the brief moments between clients, taking the first few sips of coffee or the three bites of lunch that will be our only meal in an eight- or twelve-hour shift. We can start with one mindfulness practice, incorporate it into our routine, then another, and another, eventually weaving those three breaths or three minutes of presence into a life that is remarkably free of anxiety and internal stress. If you are a runner, a painter, or do any activity in which time disappears, you know the feeling of flow. We can bring this flow into our workday as well.

Mindfulness practices can reliably bring us to that sense of an unobstructed life. Obstructions always arise, of course, but once we have trained ourselves in how to enter the full experience of the present moment, we are able to flow, like water, around or over potential difficulties, and even penetrate straight into their heart. You know the experience of suddenly saying something without any idea why you are saying it, and it turns out to be just what was needed? It's like that. You know the experience of catching a pen that is rolling off the table before your mind registered that it was rolling? It's like that. You know the experience of walking into an exam room and knowing immediately that this kid needs antibiotics? It's like that. Mindfulness can restore us to the person who was curious and connected, who took joy and pleasure in their chosen profession.

This book is divided into eight chapters.

- The first chapter explores how the regular practice of mindfulness and meditation can be helpful to healthcare professionals of all kinds. It summarizes the research on the many benefits of mindfulness-based interventions (MBIs) for doctors, doctors in training, nurses, and first responders—research that I hope is helpful for caring professionals of all kinds.
- The second chapter helps us better understand our inner critical voice and how it can sap the enjoyment from our days, replacing it with anxiety and depression. I share exercises for recognizing the Inner Critic and transforming it into a force for good.
- The third chapter offers insights into why meditation is so very helpful in restoring the health of our body-heart-mind complex.
- The fourth chapter contains mindfulness practices for connecting with yourself, the person we most often neglect as we care for others.
- The fifth chapter contains practices for enhancing your connection to your patients and their connection to and trust in you.
- The sixth chapter contains guided meditations that many healthcare workers have found to be beneficial.
- The seventh chapter offers Rescue Remedies for times of urgent need. These are very short practices you can try in the moments when emotions like anxiety or the churning mass of thoughts in your mind are overwhelming your ability to be present and to move forward with ease and

kindness. These remedies are like brief CPR that brings a sinking patient—you, in this case—back to life in just a few minutes.

- The eighth chapter includes practical suggestions for creating a group to support healthcare professionals and first responders and for designing a weekend retreat.
- At the end of the book, I have included references, notes, resources, and additional readings relevant to each chapter, in case you are interested in the research that supports the benefits of mindfulness.

You don't have to read this book from front to back. You can pick a section to read and a practice to try according to your current interest or need. You can try one practice for a week or a month at a time. You may love some practices and return to them over and over as part of your routine. Some practices may not work for you at all, and that's OK.

Many of the healthcare professionals who join our Mindful Medicine group have said that incorporating mindfulness and meditation into their daily lives has saved their careers and restored them to health so that they could return to work in the realm of human suffering, stubbornness, and courage with renewed interest and enthusiasm. These practices continually inspire and support me in finding satisfaction in my work and in my whole life.

I pray that this will be true also for you.

1

BENEFITS OF MINDFULNESS FOR
HEALTHCARE PROFESSIONALS

Why would a healthcare professional take time to practice mindfulness? Practicing mindfulness and meditation can help us become more resilient, more satisfied with our work, less likely to make errors, and make us and our patients and clients happier.

I began meditating in the 1970s, but I kept quiet about it after I discovered that other doctors considered it "woo-woo," a hippie pastime. I found two other medical residents and one nurse in the hospital who had meditation practices, and we would whisper as we passed in the hallways, "How was your retreat?"

It is immensely gratifying to live long enough to go from being considered weird to being seen as a pioneer, to becoming part of the mainstream, now so mainstream that there is a growing body of research confirming the benefits of mindfulness and meditation not only for the general population but also for healthcare workers in particular. Bringing mindfulness to aspects of daily life is a vital aspect of many spiritual traditions, including the Christian, Muslim, Jewish, Hindu, and Buddhist faiths. However, mindfulness can become a beneficial support to anyone's life, secular or religious. As Dr. Jon Kabat-Zinn reminds us, isn't it important to "show up for our life" so that we truly experience all of our remaining days?[1]

Much of the impetus to offer mindfulness-based interventions (MBIs) to doctors, nurses, and healthcare professionals in training has come from alarm about our high rates of suicide, depression, burnout, and general dissatisfaction with our chosen profession. However, in the medical profession, we demand evidence that an intervention is beneficial, especially if it asks us to take time out of an already jam-packed day.

A systematic review of research in 2020 assessed the impact of mindfulness-based interventions (MBIs) for doctors.[2] It showed positive effects in several important domains. The benefits were most apparent in programs that involved groups of healthcare professionals meeting in person (rather than web-based events or smartphone apps). Group events allowed doctors—who can be especially isolated solo practitioners—to reflect, share experiences, and be reassured that they were not alone in their difficulties. Even though we are in the midst of people the entire day, healthcare work can be a profession of profound loneliness.

The positive effects of mindfulness-based interventions for doctors that were consistent across different studies included these three domains: improved psychological well-being, improved interpersonal skills, and improved occupational well-being.

IMPROVED PERSONAL PSYCHOLOGICAL WELL-BEING

Mindfulness-based interventions for healthcare professionals reduced anxiety, stress, and worry, and improved mood, resilience, and quality of life. They also increased self-understanding and an overall sense of well-being. The authors of the review concluded that "doctors recognized that practicing mindfulness met unfulfilled needs to reflect and care for themselves."

It is not fun to drive to work with a feeling of dread or anxiety. It is not healthy to come home from work with the thought, "Did I accomplish anything worthwhile today?" Or, "I can't wait to have a drink." Or, "I just don't think I can go on like this."

Over-the-counter remedies to numb out or distract from these feelings such as alcohol or other substances, video games, sex, pornography, drugs, gambling, shopping, and eating all have the potential to become addictive—so addictive that medical people can put their patients, families, and careers in jeopardy. A respected doctor at our hospital spent so much time on a computer in a cubicle in the ER that staff complained. Then someone discovered that he had been watching pornography. Another doctor was arrested a few blocks from the hospital, on a street where prostitutes gather, when he solicited sex from an undercover police officer. I don't know what he told his spouse when his vehicle was impounded. The wife of a local anesthesiologist called 911 when he stopped breathing. Investigators discovered that he regularly came home from work, went into his office, started his own IV, and injected morphine.

Dangerous activities can also serve as over-the-counter remedies because an adrenaline rush briefly dissolves your worried thoughts and wakes you up to the vivid joy of the present moment. One of our young medical examiners took up the sport of BASE jumping. Despite warnings from his older colleagues (who had seen the fatal results of this sport on the autopsy table), he persisted and died when a wind gust smashed him against a cliff.

Over-the-counter remedies are "for temporary relief of pain. If symptoms persist, contact a doctor." What if you are the doctor? Then it's time to really contact yourself-the-doctor, at a deeper level. Time to recognize your symptoms and your diagnosis and undertake treatment at a deeper level. We hear, "Physician heal thyself." With mindfulness and meditation, that's possible.

We are not good at diagnosing ourselves. I once watched a spreading rash on my arm for two weeks before suddenly realizing, "If I saw this on a child, I'd know it was impetigo!" Another time, I dripped thick snot and had frontal headaches and low-grade fevers for two weeks before realizing I had sinusitis. Denial. We had to have a good measure of denial to go through medical training without suffering the crippling anxiety that we—or our children—had contracted every disease we saw.

We're not good at treating ourselves either. How many times have we told patients, "Take all of these antibiotic tablets," and not done that ourselves? Hubris. It comes down to not being able to admit that we too are human, subject to sickness, old age, and death. An experienced pilot told me that doctors who fly their own planes are the worst pilots and take the most risks because they believe they cannot die. Until they begin contemplating suicide . . . or other drastic measures to step back from the intense pace of our work. An exhausted doctor once confessed to me, "I had the thought that if I had another baby, I could take a few weeks off for maternity leave." Another told me, "I caught myself thinking, *Maybe if I get cancer, I can take a break.*" Thoughts like these are desperate internal cries for help.

The healing balm of mindfulness and meditation, when first applied, enables us to take a look inside and recognize our own mortality, anxiety, depression, uncertainty, and loneliness. In

Mindful Medicine groups, we can talk with other professionals about the patients we will never forget, the mistakes we will never forgive ourselves for. We can take off the mask of the all-knowing, never tiring, and unfailingly compassionate being and can be vulnerable for a change. Everyone who comes to our Mindful Medicine groups and admits to other medical professionals what has been "stuffed down inside" says it is a huge relief. And the healthcare workers who hear these confessions say that it is a huge relief to know that others are feeling the same way.

IMPROVED INTERPERSONAL SKILL

Back to the research: mindfulness-based interventions improved doctor-patient relationships through skills—learned skills—in attentive and reflective listening and through increases in empathy, compassion, and the ability to see a patient's perspective.[3] Improving your connection with your patients increases compliance with treatment recommendations, improves patient satisfaction, and can make you feel better about each encounter.

We often enter a consultation room with concerns about the previous patient(s) still swirling in our minds. We begin to form a diagnosis before the new patient has told us all their symptoms. We do a perfunctory exam because our minds have moved ahead and are already choosing the appropriate treatment or referral. With mindfulness training, we can become aware that our mind has jumped quickly into the future and we have stopped truly listening, truly seeing.

We can slow down, open into the present, and drop into absorptive and reflective listening. Then we might hear the catch of grief in their voice, inquire, and discover that a patient has just lost their spouse. Or we can notice our distracted state, look up from the computer, switch to attentive looking, and suddenly notice the bruises on a patient's wrist or an early melanoma, or catch a wince of pain or a flicker of sadness as it crosses a patient's face.

One study found that patients also noticed the benefits of enhanced interpersonal skills in their interactions with mindful practitioners.[4] If we are happier and our patients are happier, this double benefit makes mindfulness worth investigating!

IMPROVED OCCUPATIONAL WELL-BEING

Mindfulness-based interventions also reduced symptoms of burnout while increasing experiences of dedication and empowerment at work and satisfaction with a chosen specialty.[5]

We all went into caring professions with a motivation to reduce human suffering. Medicine was a calling, an honor, a sacred service we gave our lives over to. However, somewhere around 2 a.m. in a forty-eight-hour workday when we were sicker than the patients we saw in the ER, or when we got called away once again from our child's birthday party or crucial swim meet, or when we worked three weekends in a row, we lost track of our enthusiasm and dedication.

After an angry-patient encounter or hearing about a potential lawsuit, we begin to wonder, *Am I actually making a difference?* or *I'm not sure this is all worth it.* Maybe these feelings were temporary, or maybe they grew on us, until we began to feel we had chosen the wrong profession.

We all worry about making mistakes because mistakes can cost a patient their limbs or their life. Our professions are almost unique in that respect. (See the section on the Inner Critic to see how this fact feeds our inner judgmental voice and subsequent burnout.) Training in mindfulness has the potential to reduce medical errors. A Stanford survey of over six thousand physicians found that doctors with symptoms of burnout were more than twice as likely to report making a medical error in the previous three months. The incidence of medical errors tripled in units where doctors had high rates of burnout, even if the units had high safety ratings.[6] A pilot study of nurses showed the same reduction in medical errors following mindfulness training.[7]

We all work under protocols designed to reduce errors, but effective reduction may depend more upon reducing burnout among medical professionals than on up-to-date protocols. In my hospital, about three months after intensive training on new protocols for reducing wrong-limb surgery, we had a wrong-limb surgery. I swear this is true.

MAKING TIME

If research is so compelling that mindfulness-based interventions can benefit healthcare professionals so profoundly, why don't we all know about them and practice them? The most commonly cited obstacle to training in mindfulness is lack of time. Most mindfulness-based interventions follow the "classic" model of Mindfulness-Based Stress Reduction (MBSR) programs. MBSR programs, pioneered in the United States by Jon Kabat-Zinn, require a 2- to 2.5-hour session once a week for eight weeks plus a full-day silent retreat. This is a lot of time for anyone to devote to self-care—especially if they are new to the concept of mindfulness and have a demanding job, a family, religious or community activities, or even one hobby. We know how busy we are! If asked to take on a new responsibility, I can truthfully say without a hint of sarcasm or martyrdom, "I only have free time between midnight and 5 a.m."

But we don't have to carve out hours for practice to find benefit in mindfulness training and practices. The review study mentions that "residents reported that brief exercises, such as mindful breathing, were applicable in daily practice as they could be purposefully used in advance of a stressful situation (e.g., before performing an operation)."[8] I discovered this, too, and this is precisely why *Mindful Medicine* contains a variety of brief practices that easily fit into the activities of a workday. I call them practices because to become skillful in various forms of mindfulness, we have to practice them, over and over, just like the skill we develop in tying surgical knots, drawing blood, easing a big baby out of the birth canal, doing a spinal tap, assessing tympanic membranes or levels of consciousness, extracting an impacted tooth, talking a client out of suicide, or using a whirling saw blade to cut just the right amount off a femur for a knee replacement.

We all have to breathe and walk, and we can easily bring curiosity and investigation to those acts. Most healthcare professionals and first responders have to touch patients and can add the balm of loving kindness to that touch. We all ask questions of our patients and can easily add one more question that can open up an unexpected source of connection with them. We all can learn to eat at least our first few bites with the best seasoning of all—full attention to the sensations in our mouth. Many of us have to travel to work, and we can change the flavor of that often-harried commute by doing loving kindness practice.

We all have difficulty clearing the worries of the day out of our minds before we fall asleep, and there are mindfulness practices to help with that, too.

Mindfulness needn't take a lot of time but it can take away a lot of stress and add more contentment and satisfaction to our work. Over many years, I found that the time I spent in small moments of mindfulness through the day, plus the time I spent meditating each morning five days a week (typically twenty-five to thirty-five minutes), was paid back twofold during the day because I was more clear-minded, in a better mood, and more efficient. But you will have to prove that for yourself.

2

THE INNER CRITIC IN MEDICINE AND IN LIFE

The Inner Critic is a name for the voice inside your mind that criticizes you. It seems to have only one job: to point out your flaws. When your mind passes judgment on other people or anything outside of you, like a coworker, politician, or symphonic orchestra, we call this voice the Outer Judge. It's the same energy, just pointed in different directions. It's helpful to give this voice a name, which begins the vital process of separating ourselves from it so it does not make our life miserable and prevent us from enjoying our career and benefiting many people.

The Inner Critic is especially strong among many healthcare workers, and also among first responders. Why?

Because our professions are unique. If we make a mistake, we can permanently injure or even kill someone. There are very few occupations in the world in which mistakes have such dire, unforgettable—and maybe unforgivable—consequences. In our Mindful Medicine retreats, we do an exercise called "The Patient I Will Never Forget." Medical people know immediately who that person, lurking in the dim corners of their mind, is. It's never the funny or cute patient—it's the one we killed or almost killed.

It's very important to recognize the Inner Critic and to talk openly about our regrets, our mistakes, and the patients we will never forget. If we don't, and our Inner Critic is strong and unrelenting, we are in danger of becoming so unhappy that we quit medicine early or even add to the statistics of the high suicide rate among healthcare workers.

Inner Critical voices come in three strengths. The mild Inner Critic says, "Oops, we made a mistake. Well, that's how we learn in life. Let's go back and do what's needed to clean it up or straighten it out. I think we need to apologize." The medium strength Inner Critic says, "That was really stupid. Remember, you made the same mistake three years ago in March!" (The Inner Critic keeps a filing cabinet.) "What an idiot! *Don't do it again!*"

The strong Inner Critic says things like, "You are hopeless. Your family, your patients, and the entire world would be better off without you. You should never have been born." The Inner Critic is often responsible for imposter syndrome, which reportedly affects up to 70 percent of people at some time in their life.[1] "You're just pretending to be a doctor/nurse! It was a fluke you got this position. You're not really qualified to do this job." We sometimes call the strong Inner Critic a "Killer Critic" because it can literally kill all the joy in your life, and even kill you.

It is possible to disentangle from the Inner Critic and eventually transform it into a beneficial force. I'm going to give some pointers in this chapter, but getting perspective on a strong inner voice and separating from it often require outside help, for example, with a therapist. I learned what I know, practice, and teach about the inner critical voices from two interesting processes called Voice Dialogue and Voice Therapy.[2] If you want to learn more about working with the Inner Critic, see the references section for those and other resources.[3]

WHERE DID THE INNER CRITIC COME FROM?

Stop and think. Do you remember the first time you were scolded, called names, or bullied? That was the birth of the Inner Critic. There is a poignant video of adults being interviewed by a stranger about the most painful thing they were ever told. As you listen, you can hear the Inner Critic and see how long it has held on to what people were told in childhood or as young adults.[4]

To disentangle from the Inner Critic, it is very important to step back and get some perspective on it. Here are some questions to help you begin your investigation:

- Is your inner critical voice male, female, both, or neither?
- Does its voice and words resemble anyone you knew in childhood? A parent or teacher?
- What are its domains of concern and influence? For example, does it criticize your body, your memory, your work in healthcare, your relationships at home, your diet, how you take care of your own health, your spiritual life, or your very worth as a human being?
- What are its favorite expressions? Hint: The Inner Critic likes to speak in absolutes such as "you never," "you always," or "you are too . . . " It also likes to talk about "must," "should," or "shouldn't."
- Does the Inner Critic have names it calls you? Where in your life did those names come from?

WHY DID THE INNER CRITIC FORM?

The Inner Critic formed when we were quite young, when adults or other kids told us there was something wrong with us. It might have been a schoolyard or neighborhood bully, or a scolding teacher, or an angry or verbally abusive parent. These incidents tell us that who we are is defective or shameful and, if we don't watch out, we will be in danger of being hurt again or of being cast out of the social group, classroom, or family.

Unfortunately, social media has added to the power of the Inner Critic by providing children and teens with endless photoshopped images of idealized bodies and a barrage of online tutorials about attaining perfect hair and makeup.

Thus, an inner "voice" forms that keep reminding us to "watch out." It tells us what to do or not to do to stay safe. Its motives are good: to keep us safe, loved, and successful in life; however, its means of accomplishing these vital goals can be primitive, neurotic, self-defeating, and even cruel. It uses the preemptive strike, believing that if it yells at us enough, we will avoid saying or doing something that others might criticize. In doing so, it can be much more unkind than the "others" that it fears.

It is important to know that the Inner Critic is a voice that formed very early in our life, when we had almost no power and very few strategies for dealing with distress. What do small children do when they are stressed and afraid? Yell and have a temper tantrum. Yelling is a basic and primitive strategy of the inner critical voice. (Withdrawing and shutting down are also coping strategies of young children. This can also happen to people with strong Inner Critics that warn them not to talk or be noticed.) Over time, however, it can become more sneaky and subtle. It can say things like, "Other people think you are kind and have integrity, but I know you from the inside. You aren't really a compassionate person." Or "I'm totally objective in my assessment of you. Anyone who knows who you are on the inside would agree with me."

THE COMPANIONS OF THE INNER CRITIC

There are two other aspects of our inner life and internal dialogue that work in concert with the Inner Critic. We can call these the Perfectionist and the Pusher. The Perfectionist looks around for examples of perfection in our realms of aspiration and sets the internal standards for success. For example, if we wish to be more compassionate, the Perfectionist might pick the Dalai Lama, who says, "My religion is compassion," as the standard to live up to. In medicine, we might pick an actual person in our field, like a brilliant surgeon or a popular family practitioner. Or we might invent the ideal in our minds, someone who is untiring and always upbeat, loved by all their patients, unfailingly accurate in their diagnoses, 100 percent successful in all treatments, up-to-date on the latest research, actually does the latest research and publishes articles in their spare time, is skillful in negotiating with administrators, and always gets five stars on social media reviews.

The Pusher is the part of us that tells us what we have to do and the rules we have to follow in order to accomplish the (often impossible) goals that the Perfectionist has set. It is the internal force that propels us to attend conferences, read journals, apply for grants, learn new skills, stay late to finish charting, and work on weekends when we are not on call. The Pusher makes our to-do lists, crosses off two items at night, and adds four more. An unbalanced Pusher constantly adds tinder to the bonfire of burnout.

Meanwhile, the Inner Critic is the one who stands ever ready to castigate us when we do not meet the (impossible) standards of the Perfectionist or the (impossible) workload of the Pusher. This adds logs to the fire and can turn it into a conflagration.

It is not possible to get rid of these three forces in our lives. Without them, you would never have gotten through your training. They can bring tremendous benefit and happiness to our lives. However, when they are out of control, they can make us feel so trapped and hopeless that we quit the profession that we felt called to and spent so many years accomplishing. And they can become neurotic and inflated, taking up too much space in our internal world, crowding out the voices of ease, simple happiness, fulfillment, and contentment.

How do we deal with this trio? By distilling them down to their beneficial essence. The beneficial essence of the Perfectionist is the inspiration and the desire to grow, transform, and improve. The positive essence of the Pusher is determination, the physical and mental-emotional energy needed to bring about healthy transformation in our lives. The useful essence of the Inner Critic is objective discrimination and, ultimately, wisdom.

How do we accomplish this distillation? This can take some time, and some assistance. But it begins with putting a few degrees of separation between you and these internal voices in order to recognize the harm they are causing and to cease believing that they are telling you the truth.

Two of the most important ways to accomplish this separation that I have found are mindfulness and meditation. In both of these activities, we set aside the past and future and enter the refuge of present-moment awareness. Present-moment awareness is the territory outside the domain of the Perfectionist, Pusher, and Inner Critic, who depend upon shame-fueled regrets, painful self-recriminations about the past, and endless mind-spinning plans for futures that never arrive.

When our mind is filled with a tangle of competing thoughts, access to our inherent wisdom is blocked. We have all had moments when thoughts ceased, time seemed to stop, and everything became serenely clear. We call these "peak moments." Then our mind begins to chatter again, "What a beautiful sunset. I need to take a picture of it," and the moment of clarity seems to pass. However, that clarity, that serenity, that vivid beauty are always present. They are only obscured by our welter of thoughts and emotions.

Many of the most important insights in science came in moments when the scientist put aside the effort to work out a problem and let their mind be idle. Newton lying under the apple tree, Archimedes enjoying a bath, and Einstein's idle gaze out the window at a passing train led to key insights into gravity, fluid displacement, and relativity. Once our mind is clear and resting in the flow of what-is, then true inspiration, creativity, and insights can arise. It is vital to our sanity, our enjoyment of life, that we find ways and times to let the thinking mind rest and open into alert awareness. This is what we call in Zen our "Original Mind," the mind of relaxed, alert, open, and pure awareness.

GETTING PERSPECTIVE ON THE INNER CRITIC

One characteristic of the Inner Critic is that it will catch you coming and going. For example, it will criticize you for not taking care of yourself—"You can't even follow the nutritional and exercise guidelines that you tell your patients to do!"—and then criticize you if you actually do something related to self-care—"Why are you doing mindful self-compassion practice? How self-centered! Other people need kindness and compassion more than you do!" If you go to a meditation weekend, it will call you selfish for taking time away from your family or work. If you don't go, it will beat you up for being burned out and not doing anything about it.

The Inner Critic is at the heart of writer's block or any block in your creative life. It steps in as soon as you write a few words, paint a few strokes, or begin to mold a lump of clay and says, "That is pitiful. No one will want to read/see that. You are not cut out to be a writer/artist/sculptor. Give up before you embarrass yourself." However, if you do give in and abandon your artistic project, it will turn around and attack you for that. "Why did you buy all that paint and then not paint a single picture! What a waste of money!"

Once you realize that the Inner Critic is very young, very frightened for your welfare, once you begin to see that it has only one strategy for dealing with that fear, which is essentially name-calling, temper tantrums, or shutting down, you may begin to feel some compassion for it.

HOW TO WORK WITH THE INNER CRITIC

First, you have to realize when it is speaking. One doctor in our Mindful Medicine group kept insisting that she didn't have an Inner Critic. As we were doing some of these exercises, she suddenly heard the inner voice that bitterly criticized her for divorcing her husband. "What have you taught your daughter about love? How will she ever have a successful relationship?" She had an insight that the reason she thought she had no Inner Critic was, "Because I completely believed it! I thought it was the truth."

Once you are able to hear your own Inner Critic, you will be alert to its voice in others. Listen for it in your patients. "I'll never be able to . . . (stop smoking, lower my cholesterol, etc.)" "Sometimes, I just want to give up trying." "It's hopeless, doctor . . . I'm too . . . (old, confused, discouraged, overwhelmed, etc.)." You can provide the antidoting voice, first acknowledging their feelings, and then suggesting that they are being too hard on themselves. Talking about what is working well in their body or life or the progress you've seen can help, too.

Next, you need to recognize the effect of the Inner Critic. To do this, you put it in a different context than inside your mind, bringing it out into an external context. Here are two exercises to help with that. The first exercise is most effective if you do it with another person, as we do in Mindful Medicine retreats, but it can still be helpful to try alone if you are able to imagine the other person.

First Exercise

Write down more than three things that the Inner Critic says to you. One of them should be about your appearance.

Now imagine that your best friend is sitting next to you. You turn toward your friend and say out loud to them those things the Inner Critic said as if you really mean it. For example, "You are so ugly. Look at that nose (or eyes or mouth or teeth)! Can't you do anything about how you look?" Or, "You keep making the same dumb mistakes over and over. What's wrong with you?"

If you talked like that to your best friend, how long would they be your friend?

If your best friend talked to you like that, how long would they be your friend?

And yet, we allow the Inner Critic to pose as an internal friend.

Second Exercise

Imagine that you are in a grocery store. You hear a child crying and turn around to see a child cowering and the mother with her hand raised ready to slap. You hear the mother yell, "You're so stupid! Stop that crying. You're running my life. I wish you had never been born!" You would recognize this as verbal abuse. You might think about calling child protective services. Please ponder this: why do you allow the Inner Critic to say to you the hurtful things you would never say to a child or anyone you love?

Once you are attuned to what and when the Inner Critic is speaking, and once you realize how damaging it can be, then you turn toward treatments, toward remedies. Energy is just energy. It cannot be destroyed, but it can be converted into another form of energy, just as the power of a river can be converted into electrical energy, which can be converted to heat and keep you warm. What will help you transform the corrosive energy of the Inner Critic and turn it into something helpful, a force for good in your life?

PRACTICES TO ANTIDOTE AND TRANSFORM THE INNER CRITIC

Practices that fully transform the Inner Critic would fill another book, but here is how to get started. Mindful Self-Compassion, found on page 49 of this book, is a very effective, research-proven way to work with the Inner Critic. It helps to cultivate an antidoting voice, a kind inner friend. Some of the other Mindful

Medicine practices in this book also can be very helpful. For example, practicing loving kindness on the way to and from work can be expanded to include loving kindness for the frightened child who is at the heart of the Inner Critic. Gratitude practice has great power to turn the mind away from the Inner Critic's litany of what is wrong and toward the myriad blessings of our everyday, ordinary life. The exercise on becoming aware of what is working well has a similar effect.

What is the most powerful way to separate from the Inner Critic? The Inner Critic depends upon invidious comparison, upon ruminating over past mistakes and anxiety for the future. When we let go of past and future and ride the current of moment-to-moment awareness, the Inner Critic disappears. It has no traction in the present moment. Any activity in which we become so absorbed that we lose track of time—hobbies, playing with children or pets, time in nature, arts and crafts—all help us step aside from the Inner Critic. When we are able to put aside the cacophony of thoughts and enter *now* at ease within the flow of time, the Inner Critic vanishes. It is transformed into Inner Curiosity and the wonder of discovery.

Finally, if you find yourself in a situation where the Inner Critic just won't stop, try some of the mind-clearing Rescue Remedies in chapter 7.

3

MEDITATION IS NATURAL

Often we think of meditation as an extra activity, something we have to schedule time to do in a day crammed with activities. We have to put away our laptop, pull out our meditation cushions, set a timer, turn off our telephone, and then purposely engage in an activity called "meditation." We have to schedule time off from work to soak in the healing silence of a retreat. We have even added it to our identity: "I'm a meditator."

But over the course of human evolution, meditation was a natural part of life. People sat around fires and watched the flickering flames. We stood in streams and hid along animal trails, withdrawing our thoughts and human personalities so as not to be detected, merging our minds with the earth, wind, and the minds of our prey. We lay on hillsides at night, alert to sounds among our flocks of sheep, watching the stars slowly spin in the dark and deep heavens above. We walked in silence for miles and our minds expanded to include the sounds and movements of our home, a change in the temperature of the wind, the sudden silence of birds in the forest, and the slight movement of a lizard camouflaged in desert sand.

It was natural not to speak for hours. It was natural not to think for hours and, when thinking, to be able to instantly switch from thinking and talking to open awareness. Now we pay money to go to a special time and place called a meditation hall or a retreat center where we can struggle with our minds to get a few minutes or hours of surcease, of blessed relief from the endless stream of thoughts and the anxiety and stress they give birth to.

It helps to know that meditation is a natural function, one that we have lost in the rush, complexity, and sometimes-chaos of modern urban-centered life. But a natural function can be reclaimed. And if you turn toward it, and begin to practice it, eventually it will take its place again as a way of experiencing life that is the opposite of anxiety, stress, and fear about the future. This natural and most welcome way of calling up inner ease and simple happiness always lives inside of us. Periodically, meditation calls to us from within. "Let me emerge. I can restore you to mental health."

Then we make plans to meditate every day, join a meditation group, or sign up for a retreat. When the time comes to sit down on the cushion, we think, "I'm too busy today. I have to get that reading done for the talk I'm going to give. I'll meditate tomorrow for sure." We haven't yet had the experience of twenty or thirty minutes of meditation, creating a mind that is refreshed and able to do the reading more efficiently.

Or we attend a meditation group a few times, and we are disappointed that the members talk about their struggles in life and aren't manifesting inner peace and glowing auras. We haven't yet had the experience of how long-term and ever-deepening practice can bring things to the surface that need to be seen in the light of clear mind and thus become available to us so we can work with them. We haven't had the experience of talking openly to a person-of-practice about the inner thoughts that torment us and being greeted with understanding.

Or we register for a retreat, and the night before, we decide to cancel because there are twenty-three undone things on our to-do list. We haven't yet had the experience of soaking in silence, the experience of peace blossoming in our heart and saturating our whole being. We haven't had the experience of seeing the smallest things with transparent clarity, a leaf, a bowl of sparkling rice grains, dust mites floating in a beam of sunshine, or our own hands caring for us.

Because our modern minds are so full of thoughts, we have come to believe that we *are* our thoughts. Because our minds constantly plan, ruminate, strategize, and warn us of dangers, we think that the way to stay safe is to think *more*!

It is only through regular meditation practice that we are able—at will—to let go of the internal suffering that is caused by ruminating on past events—events we cannot change—and anxious imagining about the future. When we are able to rest in the flow of moment-to-moment awareness, our mental distress dissolves. We experience the blessing of a mind that is alert, but relaxed, quiet, and spacious. This is a dose of refreshment that is as necessary for our health as clean water and fresh air.

In Zen, we call this our "Natural Mind." Meditation is as natural as breathing, but unlike breathing, we have to consciously choose it. If possible, meditate for twenty-five to thirty minutes once a day. Or you can bookend the day by meditating when you arise, to prepare your mental/emotional equipment for the day, and again before bed, to clear out the residue of the day just past.

Meditate! Even for five minutes on a busy day. It will make a difference. On a day when I was rushed, I would get ready for work, dressed and car keys at hand, then sit in a chair and meditate for just five to seven minutes. Those few minutes were returned to me threefold during the day in mental clarity, emotional stability, and efficiency.

If you can, join a copacetic meditation group and find a competent, kind teacher. We all need support, companionship, and guidance in our life path.

Commit to a five- to ten-day silent retreat at least twice a year. It's like taking your heart-mind to the laundromat—you'll emerge cleaner, lighter, kinder, and wiser. What a relief!

What about meditation apps? There are tens of thousands of meditation apps for you to choose from. I recommend using an app only until you learn to guide yourself in the meditation. The problem with apps is that you become dependent upon an outside device, a device that is not always available to you in the very circumstances where you need meditation most—between patient rooms, when a procedure is not going well, or whenever irritation or reactivity surge through you.

You need a reliable inner source of equanimity and kindness that can be summoned at will. That will happen when your own mind develops the ability to calm, clarify, and expand your own mind, anytime it becomes agitated, cloudy, and contracted. This is a skill that can be developed through a regular meditation practice and engaging in mindfulness practices throughout the day.

4

CONNECTING WITH YOURSELF

To take care of others, we must take care of ourselves. And yet we don't. We know what people need to do to benefit their health: eat mostly "real" food (as opposed to food-like substances), don't smoke, drink alcohol in moderation, get enough sleep, and exercise regularly. We may feel frustrated that some of our patients won't follow these basic guidelines, but we must ask ourselves, *Do I follow them myself?*

Notice that all of these recommendations apply to the health of the body. In working with people whose bodies are sick or failing, I have discovered that a fundamental problem often lies in the mind. Here are examples. A healthy, physically fit young man with body dysmorphia was completely obsessed and made miserable by the pervasive thought that a tendon in his wrist was not attached correctly, one-quarter of an inch off what he felt was the correct site. A year after a child's birth, mothers brought in their perfectly healthy one-year-old babies for a checkup, still upset that they had to have an epidural or Cesarean section rather than the perfect home birth or vaginal birth they had envisioned. I sympathized and then tried to help them let go of their unhappy ruminations about the past and fully enjoy the presence of their living, lively baby. I had acupuncture patients who worked in "the industry" in Hollywood who suffered chronic neck pain and tension headaches from the anxiety of being called back six times for potential roles in a new movie, or who sat at home, refusing to accept a role in a TV sitcom that they saw as inferior to the role they had played four years before.

On the other hand, I have cared for children with cystic fibrosis who were happy despite their long hospital stays, frequent venipunctures, and IV re-starts. I had parents with limited financial resources, living with many people in a small apartment, who were cheerful, loved their children, and trusted in their God. I remember a mother who lost everything she had, including her house and car, to support a cocaine habit. Relieved finally to have hit bottom, she was fully engaged in recovery and had gladly taken up caring for her children again. I had a friend who had a breast biopsy. She was quite anxious in the interval before she saw her doctor about being told the results. She learned that she had breast cancer. She said that when she emerged from that appointment the world seemed washed clean, vividly alive, and every leaf in the hedge outside was sparkling with life. Her anxiety disappeared and she remained centered and calm throughout her treatment.

I realized that suffering, and its opposite, true health, depended upon the mind, maybe more than upon the body. And that also applies to all of us working in the trenches of human suffering. Although physical fatigue contributes to burnout, mental-emotional fatigue is the primary culprit. If we are to continue in our professions and enjoy it, a priority is dedicating time to the care of our minds.

I say "minds," but I actually mean "heart-minds." We are compassionate people. That is, at the bottom of it, why we are in caring professions. That means we have open hearts. But open hearts don't open only outward. They also take in the distress of everyone we see. By the end of the day, no matter how good we are at not taking on the suffering of others, a residue remains. And day after day, that residue quietly accumulates, until a soppy song comes on the radio, our parent or a particular patient dies, or we get a divorce, and the locked place in our heart opens, tears start flowing, and we wonder if they will stop.

Mindfulness is a way to care for our heart-minds without encroaching on our already limited personal time. Mindful Medicine practices can be woven into the routine of our workday. Mindfulness practices allow us to step out of the oppressive mind-cloud we call stress and refresh our heart-mind by resting in the present, even for a few minutes. It's just a few minutes, but when we learn to do this many times a day, it matters. A lot.

Here are some Mindful Medicine practices I use myself and have shared with our Mindful Medicine group that focus on how we relate to ourselves, our hearts, and our minds. We have enjoyed and learned from these practices. I encourage you to try each practice for at least a week. If you find a Mindful Medicine practice beneficial or intriguing and you want to seamlessly incorporate it into your life, try that practice for a month. Once it becomes second nature, then try another one. If you absorb these ways of being present into your daily life, it will transform your days. And your nights. And your whole life.

Wash Your Mind When
You Wash Your Hands

———

Each time you wash your hands, take a moment to invite stillness into your mind.

Let go of all thoughts and pay full attention to the sensations of washing—the sound of the water, the temperature on your hands, and the feel of the soap. You can take a few deeper, "cleansing" breaths. And, as you breathe out, consciously release physical and mental tension.

REMINDING YOURSELF

Put a small sign above the sink where you usually wash your hands, "Wash hands and mind." Or put a colored rubber band around your wrist.

DISCOVERIES

This exercise is perfect for healthcare professionals, who must wash or sanitize their hands many times a day. Research shows that nurses may sanitize their hands up to one hundred times during a twelve-hour shift. However, frequency declines over the course of a twelve-hour shift. And, even when handwashing is monitored electronically, the habit declines over time.[1] Those who do this practice report that it provides many opportunities to invest their day with small moments of mindfulness. These small pauses in the continuous stream of thoughts (often anxiety-based ones) are important. One reason we feel stressed or exhausted is that our mind is continuously turned to "ON" mode. Even at night, our brain is active, burning metabolic fuel, combining worries from the day with archetypal themes to create our dreams.

Our minds have two basic functions: thinking and awareness. Most of the time, we are thinking. You can check this yourself. Try walking down a hallway at work and letting your mind be still as you walk—gently holding it down, like an overactive puppy. Notice how your mind creeps back in and begins thinking again. It might have very brief thoughts, or quiet thoughts, but it's thinking.

This habit of constant thinking is clearly revealed when you meditate. A psychiatrist friend told me, after his first silent retreat, "If people knew what was going on in my mind, they'd declare me mentally ill." In a way, this is true. Much of our mental and bodily stress is caused by the welter of thoughts in our minds, regrets over past actions, anxiety about the future, and attacks by the inner critical voice.

We know that our bodies require rest to remain healthy. The same is true of our minds.

How do we rest our minds? Mindfulness and meditation.

You know how your body feels refreshed after even a short nap or a quick shower? You can relax and refresh your mind and heart with a short break away from thinking mode and into awareness mode. One physician discovered that this practice enabled her to "leave one patient behind so I could be present for the next person."

Mindful moments and meditation are two of the few ways and times that we are truly able to rest our minds. Taking just a minute or two to rest the mind, repeated a number of times a day, can recharge our mental-emotional batteries.

DEEPER LESSONS

A Tibetan teacher, Tenzin Wangyal, recommends that during meditation, we find a place inside that is still, completely still, a stillness unaffected by movement. Next, he recommends that we find a place inside that is completely silent, a silence unaffected by sounds. We can learn to rest our awareness in the inner place of stillness and silence. It becomes an inner refuge. In Zen, we often locate this refuge in the belly, in the center of gravity. Known in Japanese and Chinese traditions as the *hara* or *dantian*, this place rests about two or three fingers below the navel and inside the belly, in the center of the bowl of the abdomen.

Once we are centered in our body, once we are able to rest in the still, quiet space within, Tenzin Wangyal recommends that we relax our constricted, anxious mind into open spacious awareness and let it rest there, even for a few minutes. He calls these three—inner stillness, inner silence, and open, spacious mind—the Three Pills and recommends regularly practicing them during meditation so they are instantly accessible during times of stress.[2]

Snails take refuge by hiding inside their outer protective shell. When we practice resting in inner stillness, inner silence, and inner spaciousness, we carry our refuge inside of us. It's portable and always available.

Awareness is the key to a healthier life. If we find ourselves caught in a tangle of thoughts and worries, and we are able to pop up into awareness, we become more objective. We can see more possibilities and see that we actually have choices. We become free of the mind's constriction and obsessional thought cycles. Just as handwashing can prevent infection of the body by microbes, "washing" the mind can prevent infection of the mind by anxiety. Mind-washing can be a pause that refreshes and restores a tired heart and mind.

FINAL WORDS

When you are caught in a mental tangle, remember, "Mindfulness brings awareness, awareness brings choice, and choice brings freedom." Let go of thoughts and pop up into the freedom of wide-open awareness.

Just ten or twenty seconds of resting in awareness can be refreshing. Repeat often to recharge.

Loving Kindness on the Way
to or from Work

THE PRACTICE

On the way to or home from work, practice metta, or loving kindness, for at least part of the journey. Metta doesn't imply romantic or sentimental love. It is an attitude of basic friendliness toward yourself and others.

Always begin loving kindness practice with yourself. Then extend it to others. There are three basic phrases to support this practice that you can silently say as you exhale. It may help to use the recorded guided meditation at shambhala.com/mindfulmed resources.

> May I be free from fear and anxiety.
> May I be at ease.
> May I be happy (or content).

The first phrase affirms your desire—and your ability—to be free from difficult states of mind, such as anxiety.

The second phrase affirms your desire and ability to be balanced.

The third phrase helps provide a bit of uplift to our mind's tendency to focus on the negative and affirms your normal human desire to be happy.

You begin with saying the phrases for yourself. "May I be free from . . . "

As you say the first phrase, you may become aware of mental tension. Also bring awareness to any physical tension in the body, particularly in the face, mouth, jaw, neck, shoulders, hands, and belly. Perhaps that tension can soften or release a bit with each out-breath.

Switch to the second phrase when you are ready. You can imagine yourself at ease during the day, with whatever comes forward.

When you are ready, switch to the third phrase. You might notice if your mouth is tense and try letting the corners relax, perhaps into a gentle smile. You might imagine yourself smiling at some small things that will occur during the day.

When you have done loving kindness for yourself, you can switch to loving kindness for your companions at work, "May all my coworkers be free from fear and anxiety today. May they all be at ease. May they be happy."

Next, you send loving kindness to the patients or families you will be seeing or have already seen at work today.

"May the patients I will see (or have seen) today be free from anxiety and stress. (May I help them be so.) May they be at ease. (May I help them be so.) May they become healthier. (May I help them be so.)"

If anyone enters your mind—your own family members, a difficult boss, a troubling patient—you can breathe these sincere wishes to them.

If I'm short on time, I just use this single phrase: "May I and everyone I work with today, and all the patients I see and serve, be free from anxiety and fear. May they be at ease. May they experience happiness and good health."

You can change the phrases according to the circumstances. Examples: "May I be calm and clear-minded in the midst of any emergencies." "May I be kind to everyone I encounter today, including (person's name)."

Some physicians and nurses prefer doing this practice on the way home from work. They find themselves cheerful and optimistic at the start of a new day, but at the end, they're somewhat depressed and worried, reviewing and re-reviewing again the difficulties of the day. They don't want to bring these emotions home. Offering loving kindness practice on the way home or before bed can help us quickly touch on and then release whatever occurred during the day. It can also help with the tendency of the Inner Critic to disparage us for mistakes we might have made. Our Inner Critic can be very unkind to us—it can even tell us that doing loving kindness for ourselves is selfish, and it often unkindly criticizes us for not being kind to others!

REMINDING YOURSELF

You could put a sign saying "Loving Kindness" or "Metta" in your car, on your bicycle handlebars, or on your bus pass—to remind you to do loving kindness practice on the way to and from work.

DISCOVERIES

The first phrase is "May I (or others) be free from fear and anxiety."

Anxiety is a pervasive, subtle form of fear and the insidious destroyer of our happiness. It is an interesting mindfulness practice to ask the question during the day, *Do I feel anxious right now?* Check your body, heart, and mind for signs and symptoms of anxiety. The news bombards us with things to be worried about: mass shootings, stock market drops, defective airplanes, new tick or virus-borne diseases, toxins in our drinking water, estrogen leaching from plastic water bottles, new and dangerous side effects of the medications we prescribe, and the peril of high-fructose corn syrup.

As medical professionals, we are aware that while the body is the source of physical discomfort or pain, the mind is the source of people's suffering. Suffering is what the mind adds to the pain. We have seen people dying with cancer who are serene and glowing, and we have seen people with a viral sore throat who are quite miserable— sometimes because they are afraid that they are dying of cancer.

Is anxiety ever useful? Perhaps a little bit of anxiety can help get you moving when you need to finish a report or PowerPoint by morning. But too much anxiety can be crippling, and long-term anxiety can contribute to poor health. Chronic anxiety has been linked to increased risk of heart attack, respiratory distress, irritable bowel syndrome, functional dyspepsia, substance abuse, and migraine and somatic disorders.

The second phrase is, "May I (or others) be at ease."

What would life be like if we were at ease in all situations? The best medical people I have worked with seem at ease with whatever comes their way. In emergencies, they move right in to do the work needed. If things don't go well, they don't yell. They admit and correct mistakes without becoming angry at themselves or others. They are at ease and kind with patients or families who are frightened, grieving, or even angry.

I don't know anyone who has perfect inner equanimity. But a resource like metta practice is a huge help. Often, a clue that I need to do loving kindness practice is a sense of dis-ease within. I used to frequently testify in court on child abuse cases. On the way to court, I often felt nervous because I never knew how long I would be on the witness stand, being grilled; defense attorneys were likely to attack me to try to discredit my testimony. Time for metta practice. After testifying, I found that my mind would rehash the experience, critical of the responses I had given to tough questions. I would have to tell my mind quite firmly, *Enough. It's over. You did the best you could. Let's do loving kindness practice instead of perseverating about your testimony.*

The third phrase is, "May I (or others) be happy."

We are not wishing for the kind of happiness that we see in commercials, someone screaming with joy at the top of a roller coaster with fireworks bursting in the background. Rather, we are invoking the kind of quiet joy you feel in being able to lie your tired body down in bed after a hard day of work, or in drinking cold water when you are really thirsty, or in taking a shower when you're covered in sweat or dirt, or in watching someone you love relaxed in deep sleep. Doesn't everyone deserve that kind of simple happiness?

DEEPER LESSONS

Everyone experiences difficulties in life, the inevitable bruises and scrapes, or more serious trauma that can occur as we grow up surrounded by other people. Loving kindness is a natural quality within our human hearts, but it can become covered by layers of emotional armor, thicker in some people, thinner in others. As years go by, we don't realize that the default position of our heart has become a cautious guarding.

One aspect of practicing loving kindness is to check the condition of our heart several times a day. Is it open, partly open, or closed? Whenever we find it partially open or closed, we can do loving kindness practice.

No one can understand us the way we do. We live inside of us. We can hear our thoughts and feel our body sensations and emotions. No one else can do that for us. We can hope that we will find another person who will completely love and understand us and thus know how to make us happy. Forever.

But the purpose of another person's life is not to relieve our suffering. The purpose of another person's life is for them to reach their highest potential. My definition of love is this: the desire for another person to reach their own highest potential and the willingness to sacrifice what we want in order for that to happen.

The purpose of our life is to learn to relieve our own suffering, to completely understand and love our own self, and then to find a way to help other beings or other people who are suffering.

The way we help relieve the suffering of others doesn't matter. It could be collecting garbage (we would all badly suffer in a few weeks if it wasn't removed), speaking kindly to the checkout clerk, adopting a rescue animal, or helping someone pick up things they've dropped. It could be doing loving kindness for yourself when you make a mistake, for a harassed parent in the supermarket, or for those involved as you pass an accident on the highway.

I used to have a forty-five-minute commute to work. I was headed for a day of new patients (abused children), upset parents (who had learned that their child had been abused or were themselves the abusers), testimony in court with the offender glaring at me, and emergency rape cases that would keep me two hours past the clinic closing time. Doing loving kindness was a lifesaver.

Instead of listening to the alarming news on my drive every day, I would do loving kindness practice. I would do it for all the people in the cars that passed me. If someone cut me off, I'd say something like, "May you be free from whatever fear is making you drive like that. May you get to your destination safely."

I found that on the days when I did loving kindness meditation on the way to work, things seemed to go more smoothly. I can't prove it because I didn't have a control group. But I did notice how things would go when I didn't do loving kindness practice.

Maybe this benefit occurred because I was less anxious, and anxiety prevents me from feeling optimistic and at ease with whatever comes forward.

Please note that you don't need to feel any particular changes as you do this practice. People imagine that they "should" feel some physical change such as warmth in their chest or a feeling of bliss. The practice works at a deeper level and often no detectible physical changes occur.

FINAL WORDS

If you don't show loving kindness to yourself, who will?

If you don't show loving kindness toward your patients, who will?

A daily dose of loving kindness is essential to our health.

Mindful Self-Compassion

————

THE PRACTICE

Whenever you are feeling stressed or discouraged, purposely touch yourself gently, as you would to reassure a friend. You might pat yourself on the shoulder, hold your own hand, use one hand to clasp or pat the opposite upper arm, put your hand over your heart, or if you are in a private space, hug yourself. Silently say the three short phrases from this exercise, Mindful Self-Compassion.[3]

The first phrase is something like this. "This is a moment of suffering. I'm having a hard time right now." This brings mindfulness to the present moment, a recognition of what is happening right now.

The second phrase is, "It is not abnormal to feel this way. This is a part of being human." This widens our awareness into the recognition that suffering is part of the life of every person, every living being, without exception.

The third phrase calls up kindness for yourself, using words you might use with a friend or a hurt child. "I'm here for you. I care about you."

Brief, guided self-compassion practices can be found in the Practices section on Dr. Kristen Neff's website, self-compassion.org.

REMINDING YOURSELF

Post notes saying "MSC" or just "self-compassion" in several places where you will see them during the day: on your bathroom mirror, at the table where you eat breakfast, on the dashboard of your car, on your computer screen at home or at work, on your refrigerator door, or any place you might find yourself feeling overwhelmed and distressed.

DISCOVERIES

The benefits of mindful self-compassion were discovered by the psychologist Kristin Neff, who was doing graduate research on self-esteem. She found that there were problems with the popular movement to increase people's self-esteem. Rather than producing happiness, it fostered a desire to continuously compare yourself with others and a need to be better than others. It also cultivated self-criticism if you failed and anger or jealousy toward those who succeeded where you did not.[4] She began to study the practice of self-compassion, developing a scale for individuals and researchers to measure it.[5] The psychologist Christopher Germer joined her in creating curricula and training programs that are now offered worldwide. There are now hundreds of studies confirming the benefits of self-compassion in arenas ranging from A (adolescents, aging, and athletics) to W (work).[6]

Healthcare providers suffer from rates of burnout that are twice as high as in the general population.[7] We are often told to practice self-care by taking time to exercise, eating healthy foods, getting enough sleep, and connecting with friends. However, when things get hectic and we are feeling stressed at work, these options are not available. We need remedies that can be applied as we work. One of the most powerful remedies for treating burnout seems to be mindful self-compassion.

A review of fifty-eight studies of mindfulness and mindful self-compassion training in healthcare professionals (including nurses, emergency room physicians, midwives, general practitioners, hospice workers, oncology nurses, staff of surgical ICUs, inpatient psychiatric staff, and internal medicine and pediatric residents) found that mindfulness-based interventions (MBIs) had very beneficial results. These practices decreased the risk of burnout, emotional exhaustion, stress, anxiety, and reactivity. Training also increased participants' ratings of quality of life and their pleasure and satisfaction with work.[8] Many studies show that people with higher self-compassion, whether naturally occurring or as a result of training, are more resilient and are protected against burnout, stress, and loss of confidence that they are providing compassionate care.[9]

One study was tailored to the busy schedules of healthcare providers. It involved a series of six one-hour sessions offered to healthcare workers at a children's hospital during the lunch hour (with lunch provided). It showed that this brief training in self-compassion was effective in enhancing a sense of overall well-being, increasing self-compassion, and reducing secondary trauma and burnout. The program was especially successful with people who began with less self-compassion (more internal criticism).[10]

Our professions are based upon compassion, the recognition of the suffering of other human beings, and the heartfelt desire to train so that we can do something to relieve that pain. We are celebrated as heroes who put their own needs aside to continue to help others whose needs are greater. This was clear during the COVID-19 pandemic. Exhausted nurses who practiced self-compassion and felt anger toward people who had refused to get vaccinated said that when a vaccine refuser came into the hospital with COVID-19, their anger dissolved and their hearts called them to help this fellow human being who was sick or dying. How is it that our innate compassion is called forth when we see an animal or person in distress—even someone with dramatically opposing views and lifestyles—but that compassion is often not available to us when we ourselves are having a difficult time?

Maybe because we had to drive ourselves hard to get through our years of training, residency, and fellowships, to keep on going for hours when we were bone-tired and could hardly keep our eyes open, to look alert and smile as we entered each patient's room, room after room, after being on call all night or up with our own crying baby.

Maybe because we are often too busy to take care of our basic bodily needs, like eating or urinating, let alone caring for our emotional needs. We stuff our own needs and feelings down to move on to the next suffering human being who has been waiting for too long, hopeful that we can help or cure them.

Maybe because our Inner Critic—the inner voice that is the opposite of compassionate—became stronger during our training because of the risk of harming someone if we weren't perfect. The mind is so frightened when we make a mistake (or almost make one) that it can resurrect the incident in vivid detail and criticize us about it for years afterward. Maybe an administrator complained that we were "underperforming," an operation didn't go well, a patient died unexpectedly, we missed an important diagnosis and had to undergo scrutiny at a morbidity and mortality conference, or perhaps a colleague published important research or wrote a bestselling book—all of these experiences can provide fuel for our Inner Critic, which expects us to be super-human.

Mindful self-compassion helps us recognize that we too suffer. We, like all human beings, can feel discouraged, depressed, or jealous. The practice of mindful self-compassion is both an immediate treatment when acute symptoms arise and a source of readily available, long-term preventative medicine and ultimate healing. It can prevent our distress from igniting the flames of burnout and incinerating the joy of a profession we felt called to enter.

People are often reluctant to practice or even to try mindful self-compassion. We may think it's selfish. We think, *My life is easy compared to the lives of my patients or most people around the world. They deserve compassion much more than I do.* Or we think that if we are too kind to ourselves, it's a sign of weakness, self-indulgent, an excuse to be lazy, or a way of avoiding the responsibility and hard work involved in accomplishing difficult goals.

Do these reasons sound like the voice of the Inner Critic? Why does the idea of self-compassion get it all riled up? The job of the Inner Critic is very simple: it is to criticize. Self-compassion is its opposite. The Inner Critic is afraid that it might lose its hold on us if self-compassion works better than self-criticism.

DEEPER LESSONS

For many years, I taught healthcare professionals, law enforcement, and new social workers about burnout. I began by saying, "All professions carry occupational hazards. It is important to know what those hazards are so you can detect if you or a colleague are encountering them and take corrective measures. Our professional hazards are called burnout, compassion fatigue, and secondary trauma."

I asked people what they did to refresh themselves after a difficult week, what they looked forward to at the start of a weekend or a few days off. (Pause a moment and consider your answer.) Answers fall into these categories:

- Time in nature: hiking, camping, mountain climbing, and gardening
- Loving relationships: spending time with partners, family, friends, children, and pets
- Creative activities: crafting, painting, sewing, woodworking, and cooking.
- The arts: passive activities such as going to the ballet, reading a book, and going to a concert or active activities such as dancing, writing a poem, and playing in a band.
- Exercise: walking, running, biking, sports, yoga, and tai chi
- Self-care: sleeping in, napping, soaking in a bath or hot tub, and getting a massage, haircut, or manicure
- Vacations: (although people often commented that there was often so much work piled up upon return that it quickly canceled the beneficial effect of the vacation)
- Simple mastery tasks: folding laundry warm from the dryer, cleaning out one closet or cupboard, sweeping the front porch, polishing shoes, and weeding one garden bed
- Spiritual activities: attending services at a church, temple, or mosque; sweat lodge ceremonies; prayer; yoga; and meditation

I encouraged people to engage in activities from at least two or three of these categories each week. If you take your dog on a hike in the forest, you've covered three categories right there.

If people were honest, they also included these activities:

- Eating and overeating
- Drinking alcohol or using drugs

- Playing video games
- Binge-watching movies
- Shopping, including online shopping
- Gambling, including online gambling
- Pornography
- Dangerous activities such as BASE jumping, kayaking fierce rapids, and riding a motorcycle in the dark without headlights

There is nothing inherently wrong with any of this second group of activities except that they all have the potential to become addictive, and then, rather than offering relief from suffering, they become a cause of suffering.

Notice that when we are busy, most of these stress-relieving activities are not available to us. We can't drop a yoga mat on the floor of a chaotic ER or—I hope—take a swig of whiskey during a tense moment in the operating room. If we could discover an aspect that was common to all these activities, we might be able to pull it up anytime, any place the need arose.

The common factor in all the activities in these two lists is that they can bring us into the present moment. As we enter the flow of present-moment awareness, we lose track of time. When you start a run, at first you are aware of various pains in your body, but if you run long enough, you "break through the wall" into a timeless experience of flow, just breathe, step, breathe, step. Playing with young children and pets pulls us into their realm, their absorption in the present moment. Spending time in nature inducts us into the vast time perspective of mountains, rivers, and ancient trees. People often lose track of time in the art studio or woodshop, or while playing video games.

When we enter present-moment awareness, we also shed the Inner Critic. This is because the primary activities of the Inner Critic are attacking us for mistakes in the past and warning us about mistakes we will make in the future. The Inner Critic has no traction in the present moment. It disappears, and we are free to enjoy what is.

EMPATHY VERSUS COMPASSION

Recent literature and research indicate that *empathy fatigue* may be a more accurate term than compassion fatigue. Empathy involves feeling in ourselves what another person is feeling in their body, mind, and heart. Empathy is important: those who do not feel it can be callous and lack a moral compass. But empathy can create what is termed secondary or vicarious trauma. When we focus on their pain, we are less able to assist others who are in pain and even begin to avoid them. Even though we use the remedies for stress relief that are listed above, the effects of chronic exposure to suffering on our own bodies and hearts/minds are not completely eliminated, and over time, a residue collects. This occurred with me during years of listening to children vividly describe the abuse that had been inflicted on them or going to an autopsy of a battered or burned child and being unable to clear the images and feelings of what their last few days and hours of life had been like.

Compassion involves a recognition of another's suffering, which calls forth a feeling of caring, loving kindness, and a desire to do what we can to help relieve a person's pain or distress. It was the agent that called us to enter our professions. But, over time, it can morph into empathy fatigue and compel us to leave.

Whereas strong feelings of empathy lead to an inward focus, increased heart rate and skin conductance and distress-related facial and body expressions, and negative effect patterns in the brain on MRIs, feelings of compassion lead to the opposite: an outward focus, approach-related facial and body expressions, decreased heart rate and skin conductance, and a positive effect pattern in the brain. Or as one paper concluded, "Empathy (as empathic distress) can prompt us to avoid or close our eyes to curb pain caused by another's suffering. Compassion physiologically preps the body for approach and caregiving."[11]

EQUANIMITY PRACTICE

There is an augmented form of self-compassion that includes equanimity.[12] Equanimity means balance, holding two things equally, like a scale with two balanced pans. This practice acknowledges that our therapies and interactions with a patient or client are very, very small parts of the hundreds of thousands of elements of cause and effect that impinge upon that person's life. We do what we can, with skill and kindness, but we are not in control of the outcome, especially the long-term outcome. Begin by bringing to mind a patient who frustrates or exhausts you. Then read or say these words:

> We are each on our own life journey.
> I am not the cause of this person's suffering,
> nor is it entirely in my power to make it go away,
> even though I wish I could.
> Moments like this are difficult to bear,
> Yet I may still try to help if I can.

Next, begin breathing in compassion for yourself and breathing out compassion for the person you feel distressed over. This practice affirms our connection to the person and our sincere wish to remove their pain, and it helps us not take on their pain as our own.

FINAL WORDS

Become a trustworthy, kind friend—for yourself. Make self-compassion your automatic reflex when you become distressed. I guarantee that it will benefit you and your patients.

A Mindful Walking Path

THE PRACTICE

Pick a path, corridor, or walkway you routinely use. It could be a certain corridor in your workplace or the path into the building you work in. While you are walking on that path, intentionally let go of thoughts. Move your awareness to the changing sensations in the bottoms of your feet and in your legs.

Many people are introduced to mindful walking that is very slow, but you don't need to walk like a zombie down the corridor to the conference room. Walk at a normal pace or try changing your walking speed to discover how speed affects mindfulness. You can try slow-walking in a park or at home, where you have more time, space, and privacy. If you are using a wheelchair just bring full attention to the movements of your body as you travel forward.

REMINDING YOURSELF

It can be extremely easy to "go on autopilot" and forget to bring deliberate mindfulness to a familiar path. The mind tends to jump ahead to think about what will occur at the end of the path. Be creative. You could tape a bit of paper or ribbon to the toe of your shoe, where it will catch your attention or even annoy you until you remove it after you've walked your mindful path. I used to do mindful climbing, deliberately avoiding the elevator in order to climb the two flights of stairs from the hospital parking garage to my office each morning, with full attention to my legs, feet, and breath. After a week, the sight of the stairway initiated the practice.

Once you establish a path and have walked it several times, with the mind purposely directed away from reverie toward attention on body sensations, you may not need a reminder. Your mindful walking path becomes one of your "islands of pure attention" that refresh you throughout the day.

You can combine this exercise with Nature Bathing (an upcoming practice) by taking a short walk after lunch or before your evening commute. Rather than perseverating over the events of the day, direct your attention to the body sensations of walking, aware of your body moving through space, of air currents against your face, listening, opening up the visual field, smelling, and breathing fully.

DISCOVERIES

This practice is a favorite among medical people because we tread familiar paths several times a day: from our house to our car (or train station, or bicycle), from our parking place to our office, down the hall to the bathroom or the break room, up and down stairs, to a conference room or lecture hall, and then the reverse, from office to car and car to house. We can bring mindfulness into walking—or biking—without adding any extra time to days that always seem to lack free time.

An important discovery, one that is made over and over again when you bring small intervals of mindfulness into each day's activities, is how your mind seems never to rest and how much it wanders! This is one of the puzzles about the mind. Why is it not content to rest in the present moment? Why does it continually wander away from all the sensations that are happening inside the body that carries it and also away from all that is occurring in the environment surrounding that body? Why is it so intent upon going inward to the fantasy land of thoughts?

Like breath practice, mindful walking is a "staple food" for nourishing yourself when you are feeling depleted. The breath is always in the present moment. The sensations in the feet and legs as we move about will always guide us back to the refuge of the present moment.

In the last fifteen years, there has been a fair amount of research showing that regular mindful walking has important benefits. It reduces subjective feelings of depression, anxiety, stress, and brooding.[13] It can relieve symptoms of physical stress and improve perceived quality of life.[14] Research from Boston University indicates that training in mindful running and walking may help prevent wear and tear on joints.[15] It can be done anywhere, anytime, and costs nothing except the determination to hold your awareness in your body as it moves and breathes.

You can be creative with any of the mindfulness exercises in this book. Our mind often stops paying full attention when things are familiar. Driving with half attention on the mechanics of driving and half attention on the radio or an upcoming event is something we all do. However, once you begin paying full attention to what is actually happening, even for a few minutes many times a day, life becomes more vivid and satisfying.

Our human mind loves novelty, and periodically, we may need to pique its interest by changing our routine a bit. One way to bring fresh attention to mindful walking is to count how many steps you take during each in-breath and how many steps you take during each out-breath. Is the number always the same, or does it vary? The mind, especially in people who are scientifically or medically trained, also likes questions. Which part of the foot hits the ground first? Next? Last? Are both feet ever touching the ground at the same time as I walk or is one always in the air? Am I more attentive when I walk slowly, at a normal pace, or more quickly? Does one foot make a louder noise than the other when it hits the ground?

I like to challenge myself during mindful walking. I pick a certain path or set of stairs. The challenge is to stay completely present with the sensations in the bottoms of my feet without wavering until I reach the end of the stairs or my chosen mindful walking path. Sometimes I succeed and sometimes I don't, but I keep on challenging myself to be *here*, where I am actually alive.

With all mindfulness practices, not succeeding or even forgetting altogether to do the chosen practice is as interesting as doing it. Where did my mind wander off to in those few minutes? What pulled it there?

DEEPER LESSONS

Meditation masters of old compared the untrained mind to a monkey, jumping wildly from thought to thought, clinging briefly to one thought, and then jumping off to grasp another. You may have encountered people who reveal their wandering train of thoughts out loud. "Oh, your name is Sam. . . . I had an uncle named Sam. . . . he played the trombone in a band and they gave a concert every Saturday evening on the bandstand in town. . . . or maybe it was Sundays . . . he's dead now. . . . stroke . . . you're in healthcare? . . . are strokes caused by eating too much salt? . . . I love salt and I read that salt used to be worth its weight in gold. . . . I have a gold bracelet from my grandmother. . . . do you think wearing copper bracelets can cure arthritis?" You can walk out of the room and they may continue to give voice to their mind stream, with themselves as their only audience.

We can be annoyed by people with "verbal diarrhea," but once we begin to meditate and notice what our own mind is saying, we realize that we have "mental diarrhea." We just don't voice the inner dialogue out loud. And we are our only audience to that tangle of voices inside. Our untrained mind is like a rambunctious, talkative two-year-old. "Remember to get milk on the way home. . . . milk and . . . what am I forgetting? . . . watch out! That red car cut too close! . . . when I buy a new car, what color should I get? . . . red's too obvious. . . . should I get a sunroof? . . . no, too much sun. that's why I have basal cell lesions on my face. . . . remember to get sunscreen on the way home . . . what did the dermatologists say about new sunscreens in that continuing education article I read? . . . "

This endless stream of thoughts wastes energy. It tires us out. Our mind can make us anxious about a hundred disasters that will never arrive. "When an asteroid hits the earth . . . " "What if I make that error and I get fired?" "What if my son has had a car accident and is lying dying in a ditch?" The meditation teacher Mingyur Rinpoche says that to tame this wandering and keep our mind fresh and open, we need to "give the monkey mind a job." This is what we do in meditation and mindfulness practices. We train the mind to stay on one object of attention. We become aware of its habit of wandering off and are able to bring it back to the object of attention: our breathing, our feet, our hands as we wash them, a mantra, or the lovely landscape of sounds around us that has been shut out by the incessant noise of the thoughts in our head.

FINAL WORDS

Mindful walking is a job we can give the monkey mind many times a day. It helps quiet the monkey, opening the mind-door into a space of quiet alertness that is innately refreshing.

Ears Wide Open

THE PRACTICE

Open your ears to all the sounds in your environment as if your ears were giant radar dishes. Begin with the sounds in your immediate environment, and then expand your listening-bubble to include sounds that are farther away.

REMINDING YOURSELF

Put signs saying "Listen!" or a picture of an ear where you will see them. When you see the sign, if it is safe to do so, pause briefly and listen to the entire soundscape.

DISCOVERIES

Listening meditation is a very rich practice. You begin by listening to sounds that are in your body, perhaps your heartbeat or your breathing. Then you expand to listen to sounds in the room around you, perhaps the refrigerator, an office machine, or the sounds people around you are making. Next, you expand your careful listening to the entire building and finally to the outside environment.

Listen as though you have just landed on an alien planet and are hearing an unusual kind of music being played on unknown instruments. Can you hear high notes, low notes, or percussion? Can you listen as though you've never heard these sounds before? This is actually true. Each sound is just that—completely new.

People often notice that their mind wants to figure out the source of each sound and then name it. If you notice this happening, make an effort to stop your mind at one-word names and avoid beginning a chain of thought about the sound. Not like this: "What's that sound? Oh, it's a car. . . . I wonder if I should get a new car . . . maybe electric this time. . . . gotta look for a charging station near where I live . . ." Like this: "Car," and go back to listening to the naked sound. Don't manipulate. Just listen! If you do this for even a few minutes, it can clear your mind of extraneous thoughts.

Also watch for the feeling tone attached to certain sounds. The noise of the refrigerator or a siren may have a negative feeling tone. The noise of rain may have a positive feeling tone. Just notice what's been added to the bare sound, let it go, and return to pure listening. Listen to this ephemeral music—being played just for you.

It can be quite challenging to open your ears and do listening practice in a room with other people. The sound of human voices has a magnetic quality. We want to understand what they are saying. If you want a challenge, you can try listening practice at a party or any large gathering. Find a place to sit where you'll be left alone for a few minutes. Then just listen to the voices as a chorus, with sopranos, altos, tenors, and basses. My Japanese Zen teacher used to say that he enjoyed coming to America because he couldn't understand what people were saying and his mind could be very quiet.

When we are listening to our thoughts, our ability to attend to the sounds around us diminishes. You can prove this to yourself. Bring to mind a problem that you have been chewing on in your mind. It could be a problem in your family, at work, or a compelling issue on the political or international scene. Ponder it for a few moments. Now drop those thoughts and open your awareness to all the sounds in your environment, obvious and subtle. Listen carefully for half a minute. What happens to thoughts? Now switch back and think about the problem again. Then try listening to two things—thoughts and sound—at once.

We can use this inability to pay full attention to two stimuli simultaneously to our advantage. If our mind is full of the "sound" of thoughts and those thoughts are creating stress, we can clear that clutter out. We simply switch to listening to ambient sounds. For example, right now, I am sitting and writing these words, which are a stream of thoughts. If I switch to ears wide open, I hear my stomach growling, the swish of sleeve fabric rubbing as I move my arms, the tapping of the computer keys, a crow calling three times, a car passing on a nearby road, a fly buzzing at the window, the drone of a plane? Machinery? Release of toxic gas into the air? At the power plant down the river. As I was listening intently, I had to stop listening to my thoughts so I could listen clearly to the continually changing soundscape. Then all the labels dissolve and it is just sound . . . silence . . . sound . . . silence.

DEEPER LESSONS

Why does your mind want to think continually? I think that my mind seems to think that its job is to think, and that when it is thinking all the time, it is keeping me safe. Thus if my mind is not busy thinking, it is falling asleep at the inner security desk and something bad might happen to me. Actually, however, the opposite is true. It is often exactly that relentless thinking that makes me—us—feel worried. And a constant background of thinking can make us feel unsafe and chronically anxious. Does the thought "volatile toxic compounds in my air" make you feel safe or unsafe?

There are interesting questions about thoughts to investigate within your own mind and to ask others about, too.

- Do your thoughts have a sound quality—like a voice or your own voice speaking in your head?
- Do they have a touch quality? For example, are some thoughts heavier and others lighter? Are some soothing and some jarring?
- Do your thoughts involve the sense of sight? For example, when you think about a person, do you "see" them in your mind? If you think about plans, perhaps for a trip or vacation or for something you want to create such as a garden, a recipe, or a woodworking project, does your mind create images of those plans unfolding?
- Do your thoughts ever include the sense of smell or taste?

If you ask other people about what their thoughts are composed of, you might be surprised. Some people do not "think" in images. Some people do not "think" in sounds and could not tell you if their thoughts have a touch quality or weight. We constantly make the mistake of assuming that other people operate the way we do, that they experience life the way we do. The more you investigate your experience of life, the more amazed you are that we are able to communicate at all.

Here's an example: Have you ever been to a meeting in which a decision was made to do "A" and thirty minutes later you discover that another person who was at the meeting "heard" that the decision was actually "not A" or even "B"? The sound waves that arrived at our ears were the same. It was the receptive-interpretive equipment that was different.

Many experiments show how we constantly block out background noise—and yet retain the ability to hear certain sounds through the blocking of that noise, like a parent listening to a loud TV show, but hearing their baby start to cry in a closed room down the hall, or a nurse immersed in an interesting conversation at the nursing station, who alerts to the sound of a beeping IV or heart monitor.[16]

Listening practice can silence the background noise of our mind and uncover a rich world of sound that has been largely hidden. When you find your mind spinning in a hamster cage of its own making, stop and listen to the music around you. After a long day at the computer, step outside, open your awareness into the darkness, and listen to the music of the evening.[17]

FINAL WORDS

Listening to the replay of repetitive worries in your mind does not help your mental health. Listening to the constantly new and unexpected music of the world around you is much more interesting and mentally refreshing. It's a continual concert that requires no ticket.

Breathing Together

THE PRACTICE

Listen to breath sounds. After you have listened with a diagnostic ear, switch for a few breaths to coordinate your breathing with your patient's breaths. You can also do this when you are taking vital signs. Remember: patients do not know when you have finished listening to breath sounds or counting a pulse rate.

REMINDING YOURSELF

Tie a bit of colored yarn or put a piece of colored tape on the bell end of your stethoscope.

DISCOVERIES

Our breath is always in the present moment, a reliable path and guide to bring our mind back from thinking to awareness. There is a growing interest in interpersonal synchronization, the observation that people who are emotionally close tend to synchronize their heart rates, respiratory rates, and skin conductance. This phenomenon goes two ways, with the research also showing that when people deliberately match variables such as posture and respiratory rate to another person's, it can promote a feeling of connection.

When I was in medical training, we were required to listen intently to breath and heart sounds under a patient's clothing in order to be able to distinguish rales and crackles, split S2 sounds, subtle murmurs and bruits and pericardial rubs. In the last ten years, I have noticed that doctors apply their stethoscopes on top of clothing while listening to breath and heart sounds, actions we would have been roundly scolded for during our training. The extraneous noises of clothing rubbing on the stethoscope head can interfere with accurate auscultation.

No one seems to know how or why this change occurred. Is it because we feel compelled to quickly see our hourly quota of patients and lifting up a shirt takes more time? Are we reluctant to touch our patients' bare skin? Are we worried that a touch might be misunderstood? Do we believe that most physical exams will be normal? One doctor suggested it is because the information supplied by technology and lab tests was considered more accurate than what we could see, smell, and hear with our unaided senses. I found an interesting online dialogue about this question, shared more fully in the references at the end of the book.[18]

A retired general surgeon wrote, "It depends on how good you are at listening and how thoroughly you do it. To be frank, many physicians do this as a symbolic gesture to demonstrate that they are doing their job. I suspect most modern-trained Western physicians can hardly recognize rales vs. rhonchi let alone explain the significance of the difference."

An anesthesiologist wrote (tongue-in-cheek), "No, you cannot auscultate properly through clothing. It reminds me of what we used to call the orthopedic triangle during residency. An orthopedic surgeon would place his stethoscope on the chest between the top button of the patient's shirt and his neck. He would listen for a few seconds and record his results for the [entirety of the] cardiac, pulmonary, abdominal, and neurological exams. These men were giants. We seldom see their like today."

Do you notice differences when you listen over or under clothing?[19]

DEEPER LESSONS

One of our deepest human desires is for connection, for intimacy. We are born from the great mystery into separation. This is both wonderful and sad. It is wonderful that each person (including an identical twin) is unique, never before existing and never after existing in this one particular bodily form, personality, abilities, and life experiences. Wouldn't it be horrible if everyone were alike? It is variety that intrigues us and even makes us fall in love. Think about how boring medicine would be if every patient were the same.

However, the fact of our inevitable separation is also at the heart of our suffering. No one can know what is in our mind—we ourselves barely know it! At times, we may feel alienated, as if we have been placed on a foreign planet and must learn to adapt and conform.

The medicine for this dis-ease is to purposely connect. Since words can be misunderstood and can often divide, it is important to learn to connect in silence. Matching breathing is a practice that not only slows us down, brings us into the present moment, but also links us to another warm-blooded living being. When people are sitting with a dying loved one, it is recommended that they try matching their breath to the other's for at least a short period of time. Whether your patient is in a coma or awake and talking, you can link to them by matching your breathing to theirs. And, in doing so, you can ground yourself.

FINAL WORDS

When you listen to a patient's breathing, you are listening to the ebb and flow of your patient's life. And yours.

Actively Practice Gratitude

THE PRACTICE

Bring to mind at least five things that you are grateful for as you awaken and before you fall asleep at the end of the day. You could also do this at the start or end of your meditation time each day. If you do it when you are upset, watch out! You might have to give up your upset.

Try this practice twice a day for a week, or even better, for a month.

It's important to remember to do this practice when you notice your mind turning sour or your mood becoming dark.

It can help to keep a "gratitude log" where you write down what comes to mind.

REMINDING YOURSELF

Put a note "Grateful for?" on your pillow, bathroom mirror, or meditation seat.

Put paper and pen next to your bed to remind you to write down what you discover.

DISCOVERIES

People report that they notice a change in their bodies and minds after they do this simple gratitude practice. Some people notice a warming sensation in the body or chest or a widening of their field of awareness. Some report a sense of relaxation either in the body or even in the mind, which may have been holding, undetected, an accumulation of small worries or grievances.

Many people find that summoning things they are grateful for begins slowly, but once a few items appear in the mind, others begin to arise spontaneously. Don't let the mind jump in immediately with a pat answer. Let the mind be quietly open, resting in open curiosity, and see what arises.

Because the mind tends to become easily bored, after a few days or weeks, you may need to modify gratitude practice a bit to keep your mind interested. You can try categories. For example, you could ask yourself, "What am I grateful for in this room?" Or, another day, ask, "What am I grateful for about my family?" Or "about my job?"

The research on the benefits of gratitude practice is robust.[20] Robert Emmon is an expert on the effects of gratitude on health and well-being in different age groups and in sick and healthy people. Find a summary of his research at his website: https://emmons.faculty.ucdavis.edu. He found that people who kept a gratitude journal once a week for ten months (as opposed to groups who wrote about irritating or neutral events) exercised more regularly, had fewer physical complaints, fewer doctor visits, felt better about their lives as a whole, and were more optimistic about the upcoming week. They also made more progress toward their health-based, academic, and interpersonal goals. Writing and delivering a personal letter of gratitude to someone who had never been properly thanked also produced a significant increase in happiness, lasting for a month.

Gratitude practice can offer benefits even if we are ill. Twenty-one days of gratitude practice in people with neuromuscular disease resulted in more positive moods, a stronger feeling of connection to others, and better sleep than in a control group. Outward expressions of gratitude have been shown to help motivate employees and to improve partnered relationships.

One person in our Mindful Medicine group has a "gratitude buddy" to help him maintain long-term this powerful practice. Every day, they email each other a list of five things they are grateful for. The last item must be something they are grateful for about their partners. I've taken up this practice and tell my husband each night as we are falling asleep what I appreciate that he does or embodies, and he reciprocates.

DEEPER LESSONS

Gratitude practice can become the antidote when you detect negative emotions such as irritation or anger. Emotions are considered an epiphenomenon in Buddhism. That is, they do not exist on their own or arise out of nowhere. Emotions are built out of three components: body sensations, thoughts, and what the Buddha called "feeling tone."

You can watch this happen. For example, you wake up in the morning and you feel a bit cranky or just "blah." The mind detects this negative feeling tone and wants to know why it is occurring. Our mind does not like to feel that things are occurring randomly. If it can find a reason why a negative feeling tone has arisen, it can feel safer, more in control. Thus it searches through the days just past or the days to come to summon a reason, and then begins to think about what it unearthed.

"Oh, yeah, I remember that person who was abrupt with me yesterday. Are they mad at me? Am I in trouble for something?" or "I know why I feel this way. I can't figure out what to give my sister for the holidays, and the last day for mailing gifts is coming up. I really dislike the feeling of pressure and obligation at the end of the year!" or "I have too much to do today. I don't know how I'll make it through the day!"

Thus a story is added to a wisp of a negative feeling tone, and it blossoms into a full-fledged grievance. The mind may feel more in control when it digs up a reason, but in the process, we may feel more unhappy.

Other examples are the body sensations of increased heart rate and jitteriness, caused by adrenaline. Our mind can interpret this as anxiety ("I am dreading giving this talk—I'm afraid it won't go over well") or anticipation ("I'm looking forward to giving this talk—I found some exciting new research!").

One way to interrupt descent down the pathway to afflictive emotions, complaints, and grievances is to simply notice the negative feeling tone and the accompanying body sensations, without adding an internal story, even one that the mind whispers. This ability, to drop into pure sensation without any thoughts, requires a fair amount of meditation experience. Gratitude practice is a practical alternative. It can be summoned when you first detect a negative feeling tone, before a story is concocted and creates a full-fledged negative emotion and agenda to support it.

It is important to understand that gratitude practice is not a way of bypassing real difficulties. Our human mind is programmed to pay attention to the negative, the things that threaten our survival, and it often lets the positive aspects of our life drift by quickly. Gratitude practice helps us bring balance back to the focus of our mind and bring happiness and enjoyment back into our hearts. In the teaching of mindful self-compassion, this is called "savoring" what is good.

FINAL WORDS

Gratitude practice is a nonpharmaceutical way to improve mood, well-being, and physical health. It is a remedy that has only positive side effects. Try it yourself first!

Then you might experiment with asking patients to tell you one or two things in their life they are grateful for. See: Asking about Enjoyment or Blessings, page 166).

Continuous Prayer

___

THE PRACTICE

As you go through your day, try saying a silent prayer or earnest wish for the things and people you encounter.

For example, as you walk, you might pass the nurses station or your receptionists' desk and silently say to the people there, "May you all be healthy and content." Walking on a sidewalk, "May the people who laid this walk be happy and well." As you open a door, "May everyone who enters this door be well in body and in mind." As you walk past a tree, "May you thrive and provide shade and oxygen for many beings." As you drink coffee or tea, "May all those who grew and brought this coffee/tea to me be well-nourished and safe."

No one can continuously maintain this practice for a day. Inevitably, there will be gaps, many distractions, and interruptions. However, we found that as we remembered and returned to this practice several times a day, we began finding new "subjects" and opportunities for prayer or heartfelt wishes. Then the practice became more available, integrated, and continuous.

REMINDING YOURSELF

Put notes saying "Prayer" or "Earnest Wish" in places where they will remind you to do this practice. It may help to pick a path and decide from here to there you will do continuous prayers for everything you encounter. Then pick the next path of prayer. Or pick a time interval—perhaps a specific hour of patient care or during your commute home—and endeavor to offer prayers for everything and everyone you see during that hour.

DISCOVERIES

The phrase "life of continuous prayer" usually applies to monks or nuns who live cloistered lives. But mindfulness can be a wonderful form of continuous prayer. Noticing something and silently voicing a prayer, hope, or earnest wish for it is a form of mindfulness. The prayer or wish anchors us in what we are perceiving just now as we move through the ever-changing tapestry of our life. It also helps us keep an open heart.

We notice grass—"May you enjoy the sunshine." Or take a sip of water—"May everyone in the world have clean water to drink." Or read a news story or medical journal—"May everyone be able to enjoy learning new things." Or put clothing in the washer and take a shower—"May everyone be able to have clean clothes and a clean body." In a long meeting—"May we resolve all issues before us in good humor." Watching feuding politicians on the news— "May all countries be led with wisdom and compassion."

There are many kinds of prayer: prayers for help in times of distress, prayers that request what we desire to have or to have happen, and prayers of thanks. This practice has elements of all three. It can help us when the Inner Critic has taken over and is abusing us from within. It can turn our minds away from negative states, interrupting "disaster-mongering," or, as one patient named it to their physician, CTD (catastrophizing thought disorder). It can steer us toward what we desire: peace of mind. That transformation, from distress to ease, gives rise to gratitude.

For example, during the weeks when our Mindful Medicine folks were doing this practice, we heard continuous news stories about the Taliban taking control of Afghanistan. Instead of my mind creating movies of disasters with every news story, I internally whispered, "May all the Afghan women and girls be free from harm and able to continue their education. May those at risk be evacuated safely." I have no control over all the forces of cause and effect at play in Afghanistan and countless other complex and volatile situations across the globe, but I can control whether my imagination plays disaster movies over and over in my mind and makes me suffer.

Here is my algebra of suffering: If the amount of suffering in the world equals N, and seeing or hearing about that suffering also pulls us into suffering, then the amount of suffering in the world now equals N+1. Our goal in life is to decrease suffering, not to add to it. The powerful practices of gratitude, loving kindness, prayer, and mindful self-compassion can not only reduce our suffering but also fill up our emotional tanks so that we are ready to do what we can to reduce the value of N within our particular realm of activity.

Even if you begin by remembering to do continuous prayer a few times a day, if you keep returning to the practice, it begins to spread out and integrate into many other aspects of your life. One doctor in our Mindful Medicine group said that she held a fussy baby so the mother could focus on the dire news the specialist was giving her about his short life span. As the young doctor rocked him, she prayed that his remaining time with his mother would be happy and that he would feel loved. He died two months later. She said that instead of feeling helpless, offering the prayer made her feel that there was something she could do. "At least I have this to offer."

Another doctor said that her hospital, overwhelmed during the COVID-19 pandemic, had ordered a refrigerated morgue truck. She was pleased when it was announced to the staff that prayers would be offered and the truck would be blessed and asked that it be treated as a sacred space. A nurse-midwife shared that when she learned—in one day—that the director of her program was resigning and leaving the medical field altogether, that one of their patients had COVID-19, and that one of their coworkers had symptoms of COVID-19, she turned to prayers that they would all be well and at ease. That night, at her jujitsu class, she found herself praying that her training partner, nervous about her first formal competition, would do well.

It can be difficult not to carry the worries we acquire during one patient encounter into the meeting with the next patient or client. Many healthcare workers have invented quick ways to clear their heart/mind of residue and freshly come to the next person.

For example, a dentist in our Mindful Medicine group said that, as section chief for a VA hospital, he is often asked to see patients whose interactions with other dentists have gone sour. He always stops before entering the dental suite and takes a few deep breaths. This is his way of clearing what he has heard about the patient from his mind and approaching them fresh. A psychiatrist who has switched to telemedicine related that, as each patient leaves the screen, she puts a drop of essential oil on her hands and rubs them together. The smell helps refresh her for the next encounter. She realized that the next patient doesn't know that she has been on Zoom for hours. She used to be "neutral" as she greeted each person, but has discovered that smiling as she says, "Thank you for coming on. It's good to see you," makes their face light up. Seeing this makes her feel better, too.

A therapist who cares for clients who have experienced trauma, have substance addictions, and are in incarceration offered us a way of separating and clearing one patient encounter before the next. As soon as a client departs, she says out loud, "There you go . . . and I am here "(moving her hands apart in the air). "(Name of client), may you continue on your healing path and be surrounded by health and healing." She says this physical action and brief prayer supports the realization that she is actually a small part of this person's life and that there are tens of thousands of other aspects of cause and effect impinging on her client's life. It positively affects the way she feels about them, preventing her from carrying their difficulties into her own life afterward or into their next visit.

DEEPER LESSONS

It is so easy to go through a day without paying attention to much outside of our thoughts. It is so easy for the content of those thoughts to stir up anxiety. It is so easy for that anxiety to become low-level and subtly pervasive. You can try briefly looking into a mirror whenever one is available. Look at your face as though it is the face of a stranger. Does it look relaxed and content? Or do you see a wrinkled forehead, frown lines between the brows, or downturned lips? Does that face look set, worried, even sad? If you relax the area around your eyes and turn the corners of your mouth up just a bit, does that change anything in the body-heart-mind complex? What would be your prayer or sincere wish for that person you see in the mirror?

A signal that can remind you to do this practice is detecting the mind going "sour," tightening around feelings of dislike, disagreement, or stress. These are called "afflictive emotions" because they afflict us and the people around us. When these emotions make us unhappy, unhappiness leaks out and spreads to others. When you notice these afflictive emotions arising, you can immediately switch to a positive wish—what you hope will happen. This hope is what underlies your distress and is thus more authentic than your distress. Dropping into the underlying truth beneath afflictive emotions can be a relief.

You can also combine gratitude practice with prayers or earnest wishes. For example, when we notice a bee in a flower: "Thank you, bee, for pollinating and for making honey. May you find delicious nectar in this flower." Or as we lie down to sleep: "Thank you, whoever made this comfortable bed and these blankets. May you also sleep in comfort and warmth tonight."

FINAL WORDS

When we stop a moment to notice what is before us or within us and then send out a small prayer, we touch the purpose that underlies our chosen career: to do whatever we can to help alleviate the suffering of the world.

Nature Bathing

THE PRACTICE

Spend time in the natural world, ideally more than once a week. You could take a short walk during a break, eat lunch in a park, take a walk with your partner before or after dinner, work in your garden, or go hiking on the weekend. Bring mindful attention to the living beings you encounter: trees, bushes, grasses, and flowers. Open all your senses. Sit quietly and really listen. Listen to natural sounds such as bees, birds, wind, rain, or running water.

REMINDING YOURSELF

Place a small sign reading "NATURE CALLS!" or a favorite photo of a natural setting where you will see it several times a day, perhaps on your desk or on your computer.

DISCOVERIES

The literature on the health benefits of nature—both physical and mental—is extensive and rapidly growing. One of the earliest studies was done in the 1980s by a young surgeon who was puzzled by why some patients recovered from surgery much faster than others. He had been ill, intermittently bedridden with bouts of kidney disease as a child, and the view of a pine tree out his bedroom window was what sustained him through those episodes. He found that following gallbladder surgery, patients whose rooms looked out onto trees reported less pain, required less pain medication, and recovered more rapidly than those whose windows looked out onto a brick wall.[21]

Later research showed that even a picture of nature in the patient's room had a beneficial effect on pain and healing rates. Now many hospitals have installed healing gardens. Architectural firms specialize in designing gardens and give advice about "selling clients on living green walls." Research shows that connection with nature triggers physiological responses including relaxation of muscles, lower diastolic blood pressure, improved heart rate variability, and reduced cortisol levels.

Empirical studies show that time spent in nature also benefits mental health, providing emotional restoration and an increased sense of well-being and happiness, along with reports of decreased tension, anxiety, anger, fatigue, confusion, and total mood disturbance compared with time spent in urban environments with limited characteristics of nature.[22] When I was doing child abuse work, my office was on the second floor. Between patients, I would empty my mind and gaze at the tree outside my window. The changing seasons brought new buds, a screen of swaying leaves, autumn colors, and bare branches. After one minute of communion with the tree, my mind was clear and I could move on, fresh, to the next distressed child.

Terms like *biophilia, ecotherapy ecopsychology*, and *nature deficit disorder* now appear in many publications.[23] Forest bathing (*shinrin-yoku*) is a therapeutic modality that originated in Japan and is actively encouraged there. There are designated "healing forests" in Japan and Korea where people go for relief from stress, anxiety, and depression.[24] How much time in nature is effective? Researchers in Finland recommend spending at least five hours in nature per month to prevent depression, while researchers in England recommend 120 minutes per week.[25] Forest therapy has made its way to the United States with the development of the Association for Forest and Nature Therapy and its Certified Forest Therapy Guide program.[26]

DEEPER LESSONS

Human beings evolved in nature. We are a part of nature. Being separate from our original home can negatively affect our body-heart-mind complex. Only very recently in the 200,000 years of our evolution have most people lived and worked in environmentally controlled boxes and traveled around in metal boxes. We have an innate connection to nature because we appreciate the things that nature gave us to survive: food, clothing, warmth, water, and shelter. The Harvard biologist E. O. Wilson posits that since we, as a species, grew up in nature, we are biologically programmed to be drawn to it and long for it when deprived.[27] We feel at ease, at home, in nature, and uneasy—even subtly—in the city or suburbs.

Isn't it wonderful that we love the ubiquitous things in the natural world around us? Oceans, rivers, northern lights, waterfalls, mountains, cliffs, forests, and oddly shaped boulders—people will travel far to see them. They take photos to bring the pleasure of being in nature back home. In Shinto, the indigenous religion of Japan, these things are worshipped. There you will often see ropes of rice straw tied around large trees or rocks, marking them as sacred.

Ponder how different our experience of life would be if we disliked the things of nature or found them ugly. Did we evolve to find rainbows and sunsets beautiful? Did flowers evolve to attract humans as well as bees, butterflies, and moths?

When you are overwhelmed by the problems of the human world, endless wars, epidemics, and political upheavals, go into a forest and open your mind to the perspective of the trees, rocks, and the great earth. How many human lives and disputes have they witnessed, appearing, existing briefly, and disappearing? Let your tiny mind and fleeting perspective go and expand into their eternal imperturbable witnessing.

FINAL WORDS

Nature is our original home and calls us to the present moment. Time in nature may be the most important prescription for physical and mental well-being that you can write. Please prescribe it for yourself, and for your patients.

Loving Hands, Healing Touch

THE PRACTICE

Be aware of using loving hands and kind touch with patients. If possible in your work situation, try to touch each patient you see, even if it is only to shake their hand in greeting. Take a moment to make the touch a caring one as you count their pulse or palpate their neck or belly. You can add a silent prayer for their healing or imagine healing energy flowing from your fingertips.

Also use loving touch with yourself, when you wash your hands or shave. What would be your prayer for yourself?

REMINDING YOURSELF

Put a colored rubber band on your wrist or a reminder sign in appropriate places.

DISCOVERIES

We know how to use loving hands and loving touch. We use it when we handle babies, console crying children, pet faithful dogs, and touch the face of a lover. Why don't we use loving touch, or even kind touch, all the time? This is the essential question of mindfulness: if living with awareness makes our life so much richer and more satisfying, why do we fall back into old habits?

When I was in medical school, I worked with a number of physicians known for their "surgical temperament." If any difficulty arose during an operation, they would have a tantrum, even throwing expensive instruments and cursing at the surgical nurses. I noticed one surgeon was different. He handled the tissue of each patient as though it were precious. I vowed to seek him out if I needed surgery.

Often we healthcare professionals have a patient load that restricts the amount of time we can spend with each person. My daughter, a nurse in a long-term acute care hospital, lamented to me, "I want to talk to my patients, find out more about who they are, or who they were before they became paralyzed. But there's no time. I barely have time to go to the bathroom."

When we are in a hurry or upset with someone, we turn them into an object. We rush out of the house without saying goodbye to someone we love; we are blind to a coworker's unhappiness. Other people become objectified, a nuisance, and ultimately, our enemies. This can happen in medicine too and is often a symptom of burnout. "Oh, no! Not another (fill in the diagnosis)!"

When I was doing a long, slow procedure at night in the neonatal ICU, such as an exchange transfusion on an Rh-incompatible baby, I would clear my mind and pray for healing to come through my hands and into this infant. I suspect you have similar experiences of spontaneous prayer or inner surges of love for a patient. We cannot have a control group in these situations, so we cannot know the outcome if we did not pray or use loving touch. But we do know it cannot hurt.

There is extensive research on the benefits of loving or compassionate touch. Patients report feeling a difference between "diagnostic touch" and "caring touch." The latter is perceived as a sign of physician empathy and promotes healing.[28] A famous observational study of friends meeting in a café indicated that Americans touch each other less (about twice an hour) than any other culture except for the British (no touches compared to 110 in France).[29] Compassionate touch or massage activates the parasympathetic nervous system and has been shown to help premature babies gain weight and be discharged from the hospital earlier, alleviates depression and pain in children and the elderly, enhances immune function, and even reduces susceptibility to common colds.[30]

A study of married women exposed to the threat of an electric shock showed that if the women held their husbands' hand, the neural "threat response" in their brains (as revealed by MRI imaging) was less than if they held a stranger's hand or no hand.[31] Another study found that NBA teams in which team members touched each other more, as in pats on the back and high fives, won more games![32]

DEEPER LESSONS

In Japan, inanimate objects are often personified and treated with respect. Money is handed to cashiers with two hands, tea whisks are given personal names, and broken sewing needles can be given a funeral and embedded in a block of soft tofu for their final resting place. The honorific "O" is added to mundane things such as money (*o-kane*), water (*o-mizu*), and even chopsticks (*o-hashi*).

This may come from the Shinto tradition (mentioned in regard to nature bathing) of honoring the spirits (kami) that reside in large trees, waterfalls, and mountains. If they are sacred, so are the objects that arise from them.

My Zen teacher handled everything as if it were alive. I loved to watch him open his mail. Each envelope, even junk mail, was carefully slit open and the contents removed with careful attention. When we move our attention from our head to our fingers, when we touch things with careful attention—even inanimate objects—we also are touched. We establish a connection that nourishes us, too.

While doing this exercise, you may discover that you are being touched all the time. Close your eyes and open your awareness to the millions of tiny touches experienced by your body: the touch of your clothing, shoes, the chair, and the floor, the gentle touch of your eyelashes, or your two lips resting together. Try holding one of your hands with the other and imagine that you are holding the hand of someone you love. Notice that the sensation we call movement is actually a series of touches strung together and named, like "breathing." In the absence of an intimate partner, could experiencing these gentle, constant touches be enough to make us feel loved?

The person we most often forget to touch with loving kindness is ourselves. As you read this, try gently patting or stroking your cheeks as you would with a beloved child or partner. Try it each time you look in your bathroom mirror.

FINAL WORDS

"When you handle rice, water, or anything else, have the affection and caring concern of a parent raising a child."

—ZEN MASTER DOGEN

First Three Bites, First Three Sips

——

THE PRACTICE

Each time you drink or eat something, bring full attention to the first three sips or the first three bites. This means to stop thinking, move your awareness away from the tangle of thoughts in your brain, and open your mind to the rich input from all your senses. It also means slowing down a bit.

Start with your eyes. Look at the food or drink like a work of modern art. Notice shapes, colors, and surface textures.

Next, consult your nose. You might close your eyes while taking a little sniff or deeply inhaling. Coffee has an aroma, but how about your sandwich?

Now bring awareness to touch. Begin with noticing temperatures: cold, warm, or hot. The mug might be warm, but the coffee hot. You might even notice warm or cold sensations descending in your chest (esophagus) as you drink.

Include attention to the touch sensations on your fingers and hands and the touch sensations on your tongue and teeth. They might include smooth and wet like pudding, melting like chocolate, or rough and dry like chips or crackers.

Finally, you arrive at the mouth. As you take the first three sips or first three bites, bring full attention to your mouth, lips, tongue, and teeth. Be curious. How do liquids or solids get into your mouth? Where are the taste sensations strongest? Then, if you have time, try tracing the food or liquid as it moves down your esophagus, into your stomach, and soon, out to your cells.

REMINDING YOURSELF

You could put a note saying "Slow down and savor" or "First three sips" on your coffee or tea mug. You could put a note saying "First three bites" on your lunch or at the place where you usually eat.

DISCOVERIES

I have been practicing mindful eating for over forty years, and I still have to remind myself to deliberately bring my awareness out of my brain (= thinking) and move it into all my senses (= experiencing my life). When you are busy and "have a lot on your mind," it is such a strong habit to mindlessly eat and drink! Lunch is particularly tricky. It's often just a quick refueling stop. The food and drink go in while we are thinking about the patients we just saw, the patients we noticed on the afternoon appointment schedule, what we will do tonight after we get home, and what we plan to do this weekend.

Eating is one of the most pleasurable activities humans engage in, maybe second to sex. We eat or drink at least three times a day—why do we deprive ourselves of that regular dose of pleasure by going unconscious as we do it? We wouldn't—I hope—say about sex, "I have lots to do and I'm in a big hurry, so I'm going to have sex and plan my vacation at the same time"!

I find mindful eating to be so impactful that I've written books about it—*Mindful Eating* and its shorter version, *Mindful Eating on the Go*.[33] In them, I describe how I go unconscious while eating and also how to make a shift. Here's the actual incident:

I have been diligently writing for a few hours and decided to reward myself with my favorite treat: a lemon tart. A friend gave it to me and I saved it for now. I will honor the gift by mindfully eating it. The first bite is so delicious, with a flaky, slightly salty crust and a filling that is creamy, lemony, perfectly sweet and sour, and melting on my tongue. The second bite is not as intense, but still enjoyable. As I take the third bite, I begin to think about what to write next. I pick up my pen and jot a few notes. The third bite doesn't pack the pleasure punch of the first bite. I become absorbed in writing. When I stop writing, I look around for the tart, but it's gone! Who stole it? But wait a minute! The plate is still there, with a few crumbs on it. There's a lemon taste lingering in my mouth and my stomach feels full. I ate the tart, but I went unconscious and stopped tasting it when my mind moved away from its sensing/awareness function and switched back to its habitual thinking function. I became so unaware that I could have been eating the cardboard box.

What makes me smile is the irony that what took my attention away from eating mindfully was writing about mindful eating! And if I had just paused eating for a few minutes and then come back for a fourth bite, my taste neurons would have recovered from stimulus fatigue and it would have been like tasting the first bite again! It is fruitless to attempt to recreate the intensity of the first few bites by eating more, and then again more, until the entire tart or carton of ice cream is gone. Then, instead of being happier, you may encounter physical misery and mental self-blame.

DEEPER LESSONS

When we walk, talk, read, or think while we are eating, our mind is divided and we cannot be fully aware of what we are eating. This isn't bad, but it's important to observe. When we aren't present with eating, we are draining the innate satisfaction out of eating.

Then what happens? We try to summon up satisfaction by eating more! We go searching through our cupboards or fridge for something else, something that will surely make us feel satisfied. We can chase that longing and eat the miscellaneous things we encounter in our search—olives, chips, fruity yogurt, some salted peanuts, or a candy bar—until we are stuffed, but nothing stops that feeling of fundamental dissatisfaction.

Intimacy is the antidote to dissatisfaction. As this book shows over and over, intimacy is our heart's true longing. And we can find a kind of intimacy through mindful eating. I once taught the common practice of mindfully eating a single raisin to a group that included a Catholic priest. After the others left, he approached me, marveling that a single raisin had flooded his mouth with sensations and his entire being with joy. He said it brought back the experience he'd had at his first communion, when a small wafer had filled him with subtle flavors and complete satisfaction. Decades later, this was still his experience of communion, coming into union with this very moment and thus with God. This is the mystery that accompanies times of presence.

Eating is a sacred activity. It connects us to countless forms of life. One bite of the banana bread I just baked is full of the life energy of many plants: flour from rice, sorghum, tapioca, and corn; fruit from banana plants; and sugar from cane and maple trees. Reading the label on the vegan "butter" I will spread on the bread opens my mind-door to oils from more plants, including palm, canola, soybean, flax, and olive trees. The word *flax* turns my mind to the bed of flax plants we grew last year at the monastery. Flax has tall slender stems with lovely blue flowers, and when you water with a sprayer, the plants all dance in the sun! As I eat, the joy I felt watching the dance spreads into my body and mind.

If I open my awareness further, I can "see" the various people who planted, grew, and harvested those twelve flour and oil plants and those who mined the salt and monitored the chemical processes that produce the baking powder the recipe called for.[34] Actually, all food is the energy of sunlight, converted by plants and animals into a form that we can consume. We take sunlight, earth, rain, and the life energy of myriad beings into our body every time we eat, drink, or have a snack. We are quite literally sunshine appearing temporarily in the form of a human body.

FINAL WORDS

Mindful eating is a path to what we long for: connection to others and the great mystery that is our life. Even when we are in a hurry, we can briefly pause to savor the first few bites or sips, to open that connection and give thanks.

Simple Joys

THE PRACTICE

Each day, please find something that gives you simple joy and do it! It might be something you did as a child, like lying on the grass and watching the clouds changing shape, or counting the cracks in the sidewalk from your car to your office and stepping over them so you don't "break your mother's back," or stopping to say hello to the flowers or leaves that you ordinarily barely notice as you walk by, lost in thought. Bring close attention to the colors, shapes, and fragrances of these living beings who share and beautify your world. It only needs to take a few minutes.

DISCOVERIES

The members of our Mindful Medicine group had fun talking about the things they do that could be called childlike or silly pastimes. *Childish* and *silly* are words the Inner Critic uses to keep us from having fun. Childlike is different from childish. Childish implies self-centered, petulant behaviors. Childlike refers to the inherent curiosity, open awareness, and lack of self-consciousness of a young child.

One person said that after a stressful day, they pulled out a collection of musical instruments (harmonica, ukulele, mbira, and an Indian flute) that they did not know how to play and just blew and banged on them for a while. Another person confessed to talking in silly voices on long drives in their car. An ob-gyn said she turned on loud music and had a one-person dance party in the kitchen. People also enjoyed letting their childlike side emerge when they played with pets and with grandchildren.

One doctor spoke about the benefits of laughter yoga—intentionally laughing for five to thirty minutes a day—and we all tried it. Even laughing together on-screen over Zoom for a few minutes was noticeably refreshing to body and mind, a result that has been confirmed by research. Practicing laughter yoga has been shown to lower blood pressure, self-reported stress, depression, and anxiety and reduces morning cortisol levels. It results in a release of endorphins, oxytocin, and serotonin. A few fifteen-minute sessions of laughter yoga have been shown to increase feelings of self-efficacy, self-confidence, and connection to others as well as the ability to maintain equanimity and a positive outlook even in the face of disruptive thoughts and emotions. Laughter increases tolerance of pain and even provides light aerobic exercise![35]

Silly Walking is a mindfulness practice that always cheers me up. It is based upon the *Monty Python* sketch about the Ministry of Silly Walks.[36] When I notice that my mind is beginning to turn sour, I find that walking backward or skipping a bit reliably lightens my mood and turns it toward joy. There's also a website with satirical medical "news," gomerblog.com, much like The Onion, with articles like "Hospital Combats Physician Burnout with Mandatory Training on Burnout."[37] A short, funny video at night can help you go to bed with a smile.

DEEPER LESSONS

Mind training is critical to our happiness. In the spacious silence of meditation, we can watch what our mind is up to. We can learn to detect when it first begins to cloud over, even with the subtle beginnings of an afflictive emotion. The term *afflictive emotion* refers to emotions that afflict us with suffering, including anger, hatred, anxiety, jealousy, greed, envy, and lust. We might think that these emotions are natural to any human being and should be expressed. These emotions may be natural, but expressing them ignores their consequences. When these negative emotions radiate out or are acted out by one person, they can cause distress to many other people, including our partners, patients, coworkers, children, and even pets.

In the West we tend to think of emotions as arising in the heart, not in the mind, but, as mentioned earlier, emotions actually are a combination of thoughts, body sensations, and "feeling tone," a subtle flavor that turns the mix of body sensations and thoughts toward pleasure or pain. For example, if your body is aching and you add a negative feeling tone, your thoughts will also be negative. "Something is wrong! Am I coming down with the flu? Is the pain getting worse? Maybe I have something really bad, something that can't be cured!" If your body is aching and you add a positive feeling tone, your thoughts might be, "That was such a good workout! My body really needed it. I'm becoming more fit every day."

If you are angry and you stop thinking entirely, entering wide-open awareness, all that is left are body sensations, which will inevitably change and recede—if they are not fed the fuel of thoughts. It is thoughts that keep afflictive emotions alive.

Mindfulness can help us recognize what is going on in our heart-mind before it expands into full-blown suffering. Mindfulness then helps us choose among the practices that can turn the mind around before it starts down the steep chute to unhappiness. Meditation, especially long silent meditation retreats, provides time and space to become ever more skilled in detecting the subtle aspects of mind movement toward negative emotions, as well as time and space to gain experience and confidence in our ability to change our own mind. Gradually, we become free from the tyranny of our mind. We become what Zen masters call the "Master and Mistress of the House," at ease and at home in our own being.

The Buddha often used analogies involving everyday objects, whose working was familiar to everyone in his audiences. He spoke about how deep ruts form when a cart always follows the same track. If we see a cart is headed downhill toward trouble—like quicksand—and we want to arrive at a different destination—like a dry, firm road—we need first to see the ruts, then to lift the cart out of the ruts and place it on another path. Eventually, with enough practice in detecting and adjusting, new ruts will form that reliably direct the cart toward safety. This is exactly what we do in training our heart-mind.

Unsophisticated, childlike activities like dancing or making spontaneous music have the ability to pick up the cart of our heart-mind and turn it toward a quiet happiness and simple contentment that are everyone's birthright.

We spend our days caring for the vulnerable people in our community. Sometimes, that means our own vulnerable parts get overridden. They are the parts of us that find delight in simple things, like watching two ants working together to carry a big crumb back to their nest, or the way robins chirp and change the phrases of their song, or how the long sun rays descend from heaven to earth through a hole in the clouds. One day, I was striding through the lobby of our hospital and I heard two small children exclaim, "Look, Mommy, the grass is dancing!" As their mother hurried them along, they were pointing to the long grass in the healing garden outside the window. I slowed to see what their mother would do. Bless her; she stopped and then I stopped too and we all looked at the wind-tossing grass with smiles on all our faces.

FINAL WORDS

Joy can be cultivated. Please stop, look around, listen, and give the young and wonder-filled part of you a few special minutes each day.

The Mysterious Life of Your Tongue

THE PRACTICE

This is one of my favorite investigations. Watching your tongue in action is fascinating, often humorous, and directly relevant to your practice in healthcare. I'm always making new discoveries when I bring sustained attention to my tongue.

A good way to begin this practice is to watch your tongue as you eat and then ask questions. How does my tongue help get food into my mouth? Does it go under or on top of the spoon or fork?

What does it do with the food once it is inside?

How is my tongue involved in chewing?

REMINDING YOURSELF

Put a note, "What is my tongue doing now?" at the place where you usually eat meals.

DISCOVERIES

Getting food in: Our tongue is such a busy little being, and it's hard to catch what it's doing without slowing down the processes of eating and drinking. Try a stop-motion process to help you watch it. As you bring a bite of food toward your mouth, let the tongue show you, one small movement at a time, how it gets the food off the fork or spoon. Observe also how it helps bring liquids into the mouth.

Chewing: Do the same thing with chewing. Try chewing without moving your tongue. Now slowly bring your tongue back online and watch in slow motion what it does as you chew, one deliberate chew at a time.

Swallowing: The next part of the investigation involves swallowing. How is my tongue involved in swallowing? Try chewing for a while and deliberately not swallowing and see what happens. How does my tongue decide when to swallow? What are its (several) criteria for concluding, "OK to swallow this"? Watch carefully.

Advanced noticing: Does your tongue allow food to creep down the throat without actively swallowing?

After you eat: Once you've finished chewing and swallowing, what does your tongue do now? How long does it take your tongue to start resting after eating?

Advanced noticing: Is your tongue ever quiet?

Tasting: The map of taste areas on the tongue was created in 1906 and is not accurate. Discover for yourself: where on your tongue do you taste salty food the most vividly? Sugary? Spicy? Umami? Minty?

Our tongues are not only active in eating, but also in talking. Try saying something, maybe a poem you've memorized or a chant, and watch how your tongue shapes and moves to produce different letters, vowels, and consonants. Try slowly repeating the word *dot* to watch as your tongue shapes itself to make a *d* sound different from a *t* sound? Try saying "grass" and "glass" and watch it make an *r* versus *l* sound. These two sounds can be difficult to distinguish for people who are native speakers of some other languages, for example, Japanese, because they are combined into one sound in these languages. In Spanish, however, the tongue rolls a more exaggerated *r* sound. Babies learn these differences quite early, perhaps even before birth.[38]

The Korean alphabet was developed in the mid-1400s by a king who was successful in his desire to create universal literacy among his subjects. If you watch your tongue as you pronounce the sounds *s*, *j*, and *ch*, you will understand the Korean saying about this very logical alphabet: "A wise man can acquaint himself with them before the morning is over; even a stupid man can learn them in the space of ten days."

ㅅ = s, ㅈ = j, ㅊ = ch. The letter *j* is an *s* with one line over it, and *ch* is an *s* with two lines over it.

What do these lines indicate about what is happening in your mouth as you say these letters?

DEEPER LESSONS

Once you spend time watching your tongue, you can see now how severe a punishment cutting off a tongue would be. You will have an increased understanding of the struggles of a patient with a stroke affecting the tongue or surgical removal of a cancerous part of the tongue.

I like to count the many jobs of the tongue. As we eat, it serves as a shovel, a sucking straw, a guardian of the airway, a sorter, a mixer-blender, a gatherer-swallower, a constant tester of tastes, textures, and temperatures, and finally, a janitor and a toothpick. Have you noticed how determined it is to patrol your teeth, and it keeps worrying at a piece of food stuck in them until it can pry it loose? Once you watch your tongue in action, you marvel at its dexterity. How does it stay out of the way of the teeth as we chew? Or chew and talk? It can even keep us mobile when the rest of the body is paralyzed! A small magnet pierced in the tongue of patients who are quadriplegic can enable them to move about more skillfully in a wheelchair than using the traditional puff and suck method.[39]

You could not build a machine that does what the tongue does, and you could not instruct your tongue how to carry out its tasks.

"Push the food to the left side teeth. Look out! Get out of the way quickly! Here come the teeth! Now hurry up and grab some food from the teeth on the left and push it to the teeth on the right side—look out! Here come the teeth!" In fact, if you try to control your tongue during eating, you are likely to bite it.

Tongue practice is one of the best examples of the power of mindfulness. It clearly shows us that when we bring sustained attention to anything—*anything*—it will open into an entire universe. Mindful attention can turn any day, any few minutes, into an adventure. There are so many new discoveries just waiting for us to stop thinking and open our minds into interested awareness.

Our tongue is like a little person inside of us, busily multitasking, constantly caring for us from before we were born, a person we have almost entirely ignored—unless we bite it or burn it. It is part of what we call in Zen our True Nature, which is always caring for us whether we are aware of it or not. There is research showing that when our tongue is moving, so is our mind. You might try consciously resting your tongue, in order to rest your mind.

FINAL WORDS

You are always being cared for, twenty-four hours a day, by your tongue and by the many other organs hidden in your body. Like the other things in our life, they tend to operate better when we don't try to control them.

Not Touching Your Face

THE PRACTICE

For one week, be mindful of not touching your face with your hands.

Notice what happens just before the impulse to touch your face arises. Was it a thought? A physical sensation? An emotion?

This practice includes not resting your face on your hands. When you do necessary activities such as blowing your nose, washing your face, shaving, or putting on makeup, simply notice that you are intentionally touching your face.

It is important to do this exercise ourselves since we must do it when we are caring for a patient under isolation or infection precautions and may need to recommend it to family members of infectious patients.

REMINDING YOURSELF

Post notes in appropriate places around your home, office, and on your computer: "Don't Touch Your Face." Because touching our face occurs so frequently and is largely an unconscious activity, you may need to enroll someone else to signal you when you are touching your face.

DISCOVERIES

It is very hard not to touch your face!

Many people realized this for the first time when the COVID-19 pandemic spread around the world, and we were advised to make not touching our face an important practice for our safety.

Some people report that as soon as they decide to stop touching their face, they become acutely aware of many small sensations that trigger the urge to touch their face. It could be a small itch, an odd sensation inside the ear canal, a bit of dried matter in the opening to the tear duct, a piece of fluff irritating the nostrils, or the tongue discovering that something is stuck between the two front incisors and the fingers responding to help out.

People who do long meditation retreats learn to concentrate so deeply on something like their breathing that they are no longer disturbed by those small sensations. They train themselves to stay with annoying sensations, watching them appear, grow, change, and fade away. Perhaps healthcare workers in certain specialties also do this kind of training and are better at restraint. For example, surgeons in the operating room cannot break sterile technique if there is sweat running down their cheek or have an itch and may have to ask a circulating nurse or anesthesiologist to wipe their faces or scratch their backs.

A study of twenty-six medical students who were filmed while watching a lecture showed that each student touched their face an average of twenty-three times in one hour! Of those touches, 44 percent involved a mucous membrane, the mouth (36 percent), eyes (31 percent), or nose (27 percent), with 6 percent being a combination of these areas.[40]

A study of clinicians (thirty-one) and staff (forty-eight) at seven primary care clinics in the Cincinnati area revealed that they touched their T-zones (eyes, nose, and mouth) a mean of nineteen times in two hours (range, 0–105 times); clinicians did so significantly less often than staff ($p < 0.001$). Researchers also observed hundreds of episodes of handwashing and uses of alcohol-based cleansers. Only 9 percent of handwashings met the Centers for Disease Control and Prevention criteria for effective handwashing! Alcohol cleansers were used more appropriately, with 84 percent meeting ideal use.[41]

DEEPER LESSONS

We know that good handwashing and avoiding touching your face are effective ways of preventing the spread of many bacteria and viruses, but we find it is not so easy to do ourselves. It takes determination to break an unconscious habit! As one of my professors said, "The unconscious is unconscious." Only when a thought, emotion, or even an action is brought into the light of conscious awareness is there any chance of changing it.

Bringing it into conscious awareness is one thing, but holding it there throughout a day, while many distractions arise, is another. It is almost impossible to pay full attention to two things at once. That's why we need reminders, like signs. But eventually, the signs become part of the wall, and we stop seeing them.

The experience of practicing safety measures during epidemics of infectious agents has consequences. It is easy to develop aversion: to people who sneeze or cough, to shaking hands, to people standing close, to closed spaces such as elevators, or even to our own face or body. When you notice that aversion arising, try a few minutes of loving kindness practice. On each out-breath, silently say, "May I be at ease."

FINAL WORDS

Mindfulness can bring fresh awareness to each day, each encounter, and each small impulse to touch our face.

Remembering Your Vow

THE PRACTICE

Take a few minutes to ponder how, when, and why you decided
to become a healthcare professional or first responder. Write out
your decision in a few sentences or paragraphs. For example,
"When I was six, I got something in my eye on the playground.
I went to see the school nurse and she washed my eye out. She
was so kind, I decided that I would become a nurse so I could
help people who are in pain. I used to play hospital with my dolls,
bandaging them up." Or, "My younger brother contracted men-
ingitis and died when I was in college. I decided that I wanted to
be a doctor so this wouldn't happen to more kids. I was an English
major so I had to take my prerequisites for applying to medical
school in summer school."

Then condense that decision down into a short vow or mission statement for your life. Perhaps you already know what it is.
If not, here are a few suggestions: "I am an oncology doctor/nurse
because I want to give children with cancer a chance at a long
and happy life." Or "I became a neurosurgeon because the human
brain is the most important organ in the body and I am skilled at
delicate surgery." Or " I became an EMT because I can save lives
when disasters occur."

REMINDING YOURSELF

Post those short sentences about your vow or mission statement
wherever you will see them at least once a day, perhaps on your
bathroom mirror, refrigerator, or the frame of your computer
screen.

DISCOVERIES

In Zen, we talk about clarifying our personal vows. Our life is composed of many vows, some small and temporary and others larger and foundational throughout our life. Perhaps you made an inner promise to learn to play a musical instrument. You had to practice for long hours, giving up other options like joining a pickup game of ball. You had to renew your intention when you faced obstacles or grew discouraged. If you raised children, you made a vow to be a good parent and renewed that vow over and over in the face of smelly diapers, toddler tantrums, and cranky teenagers.

These kinds of vows might not be stated out loud, but they continuously weave the fabric of every person's life. Vows keep us from acting unconsciously and from being buffeted about by karmic cause and effect. They act as a conduit for our life energy, and an inner GPS, so we do not end up on our deathbeds wondering how we ended up here and whether our life was worthwhile.

Becoming a medical professional means embarking on a long training journey and giving up many other things we might like to do in life. These sacrifices continue throughout our career: not having time to eat lunch, missing holiday celebrations, and not taking good care of our own physical and mental-emotional health. We wouldn't make these sacrifices if we didn't have a strong inner purpose or vow or, as one person in our Mindful Medicine group called it, a clear mission or calling in life.

If you are part of a Mindful Medicine or another support group for providers, this is a topic that will help you discover many things you did not know about your members. One person can tell the story of their journey to becoming a healthcare professional while the other person practices compassionate, attentive listening. Then reverse roles.

In our Mindful Medicine retreats, we often do this exercise. It's surprising how often people have lost sight of their original reason for entering medicine. We can call those decisions choosing a life purpose or a life vow. The word *vow* seems like a strong word and can be tainted by the Inner Critic's attacks on us for breaking our marriage vows if we have gone through a divorce. However, we purposely use the word *vow* instead of its synonyms because it reflects our strong commitment to helping others. *Promises* are too easily broken. *Intentions* may be good, but are too easily deflected. *Oath* has a strong military flavor. *Mission* is closer, but many businesses have mission statements that begin with making a profit for shareholders, probably not our motive. *Essential life purpose* comes closer. My husband coined the phrase "the heart's deepest aspiration."

There is a substantial body of writing and research in the field of psychology on the benefits of life goals. The research reveals that humans are goal-making beings and vows are good for our life. Certain types of life goals are linked to physical and mental-emotional health, satisfaction in life, and a feeling that your life has meaning no matter what challenges are arising at this time. Those goals are spiritual (seeking greater intimacy with the divine), generative (involving creativity, giving of oneself, and serving generations in the future), and those that involve intrinsic sources of satisfaction (self-discipline, intimacy with others, and self-confidence). Life goals that involve extrinsic sources of satisfaction (power over others, financial gain, fame, and physical attractiveness) do not produce well-being and may even lower it.[42]

Research also shows that conflicting goals can become stressful. In the healthcare field, a common conflict is "keeping up on the latest research and training in advanced skills in my field" versus "spending quality time with my family" versus "devoting more time to meditation and attending retreats so I can remain clear-minded and serene in the face of challenges."

Many of us took vows at the end of our training, a version of the Hippocratic oath, the Declaration of Geneva (developed after the medical atrocities of World War II), the Oath of Maimonides, the Nightingale Pledge, the Osteopathic Oath, or a pledge authored by faculty or students. Most of us likely have forgotten what we recited.

These oaths contain common elements:

to respect my colleagues and those who have gone before
to extend and gladly share my knowledge and skills
not to cause harm
to guard a patient's secrets even after the patient dies
to prevent disease when I can
and to not permit prejudice to affect my duty to my patients.

Some oaths include unique promises:

I will remember that there is an art to medicine as well as science and that warmth, sympathy, and understanding may outweigh the surgeon's knife or the chemist's drug.
I will not be ashamed to say "I do not know," nor will I fail to call in my colleagues when the skills of another are needed for a patient's recovery.
May I never see the patient but as a fellow creature in pain.

There are some recent additions to these oaths.

> I will remember that I do not treat a fever chart, a cancerous growth, but a sick human being, whose illness may affect the person's family and economic stability. My responsibility includes these related problems, if I am to care adequately for the sick.
>
> I will attend to my own health, well-being, and activities in order to provide care of the highest standards.

DEEPER LESSONS

There are different kinds of vows.[43] Some are inherited from our family, perhaps a parent who was passionate about being a nurse, firefighter, or medical missionary. Parents who were thwarted in carrying out their vows may pass them on to their children, urging them to become doctors so they will be financially stable. Or the reverse. The father of a friend was a vigorous rural veterinarian who died of pancreatic cancer a month after being diagnosed. He told his children that he regretted how all-consuming his profession had been and how much of family life he had missed, warning his children not to follow his path.

Some vows are inspired by people we know and admire, or by icons like Albert Schweitzer or Mother Teresa. Some vows are reactive. If we grew up in an alcoholic family, we may vow never to drink alcohol or we may become addiction specialists. One female doctor said that her determination to go to medical school was boosted when her college premed adviser said, "I see you have a sorority pin. You should just find someone who wants to be a doctor and marry him." A similar patronizing verbal "pat on the head" happened to me when I told a doctor in a hospital where I worked one summer as a nurses' aide that I wanted to become a physician. In both instances, the effect was a reactive inner voice saying, "Well, I'll show him!" and it strengthened our purpose.

I have a theory that underlying many healthcare professionals' careers are reactive vows, a desire to gain control over a type of suffering they witnessed in early life (just as many people became lawyers because of experiences of injustice in early life). I thought this wasn't true of me until I remembered that at age five I had a mysterious illness with fevers, swollen lymph nodes, and fatigue that kept me in bed for a month. I remember our doctor drawing what seemed like huge syringes of my blood, the treats of ice cream afterward if I held still, and the palpable worry in the air and on everyone's faces. Looking back, I think I had mononucleosis, but I realize now that the adults were worried that I had leukemia.

As we discussed reactive and inspired vows in our Mindful Medicine group, one doctor realized that she had undertaken a thirteen-year training program in neurodevelopmental disorders partly because she had grown up with an uncle who had cerebral palsy. When I asked a psychiatrist about any early experiences with mental illness, she recounted that her great-uncle had bipolar disorder, her father had seizures, and both her parents lived with depression and benefited from medication.

Can you see the action of inspired vows and reactive vows in their stories? Can you detect these forces acting in your decision to enter a healthcare profession?

It is important not to confuse the means—the current way to accomplish your vow—with your vow. Your current means might be serving as a family practitioner or a dentist, but when you retire from that profession, your underlying vow doesn't retire.

If you know what your vow is, perhaps to help relieve unnecessary human suffering, you can easily find another means, maybe volunteering in a clinic for seasonal migrant workers or mentoring struggling medical students or joining a mission to a country that has experienced a violent earthquake.

FINAL WORDS

Life is the primary vow. Without life, no other vows are possible. Our work enables us and those we serve to carry out vows that, over time, will bring benefit to countless people and other beings.

Working with Anger

THE PRACTICE

Notice when you are becoming angry. Pay attention to the body sensations that signal, "Anger is arising." When you are able, investigate these questions.

- Are there certain people or situations that I often react to with anger?
- If I got angry and spoke or acted from anger, did it help the situation or make it worse?
- Can I find a fear underneath that anger?

REMINDING YOURSELF

Wear a red wristband, and each time you discover that you are getting irritated or angry, move it to the other wrist. Then try at least one of the brief practices at the end of this chapter.

DISCOVERIES

Sometimes, we get angry—at patients, at coworkers, at the head of our division, or "the administration." Sometimes, we get angry at people we love. Sometimes, we get angry at ourselves.

Anger is such a common problem that we held a series of classes on anger at the monastery where I live. We began by asking these questions:

- How do I know I'm angry? What are the first signals that alert me to the arising of anger?
- Is anger ever helpful or beneficial?

- Does expressing anger in speech or action ever have a good outcome or does it do more harm than good?
- Is there anything that consistently provokes anger in me?
- What is the ultimate source of anger? If we know the source, we can find a treatment.

We discovered that everyone has different body signals that herald the appearance and growth of anger. Some people notice an increase in heart rate and a tightening in their chest. Others report that their jaw clenches and their hands fold into fists, or their eyes narrow and their faces flushes. It's important to know what you feel in your body when you begin to get angry.

Why? Because it's an early warning signal that anger is arising. Anger occurs on a spectrum, from impatience to irritation through annoyance, exasperation, anger, fury, and murderous rage. When, through mindful awareness, we catch anger early, then we have a choice about what to do with it. And that choice can either lead us deeper into anger and its consequences or open a door into dissolving anger and transforming its power into a force for good.

Is anger ever helpful or beneficial? Endless injustice in the world could make us angry enough to "fuel a mission" and take up a cause such as sex trafficking, child abuse, climate change, racism, world hunger, and war. The world is full of problems, and we have a choice. We can either work to change these problems from an inner place of equanimity or from a place of anger, which only adds to the anger in the world, particularly if we try to get agreement about our anger and gather more people around this feeling. Anger can be an effective *messenger* that something is wrong, but is not an effective *means* to solve that wrong. Maybe our own anger is the only thing we can change.

Anger is often an unpleasant feeling, and also an expensive fuel—one that takes a toll on our bodies. It can make us feel off-balance, even out of control. It also tends to create "the other side" and make those people angry, too. But, as one participant in the monastery's course on anger commented, "Sometimes, anger is delicious because I feel so righteous."

Anger can bring the energy necessary to tackle a wrong, but first, it must be transformed from the reactive energy of anger into the productive energy of great determination. Models of great determination in loving action are present across time, culture, and traditions and include Greta Thunberg, Mahatma Gandhi, Mother Teresa, Albert Schweitzer, the Dalai Lama, Martin Luther King Jr., and Thich Nhat Hanh.

DEEPER LESSONS

I am writing this amid the fourth surge of COVID-19 cases in the state where I live—the worst so far—with a shortage of ICU and regular hospital beds, staff shortages, and refrigerated morgue trucks. Anger seems to be invading medical care, in our state and other places where COVID-19 is surging. Anger related to the COVID-19 pandemic and how people have responded makes sense. Healthcare workers face myriad challenges—from belligerent patients and families who refuse best practices in medical care because of belief in conspiracy theories to staff shortages heightened by colleagues quitting in burnout or in response to a vaccine mandate. Yet, anger in healthcare was present even before the pandemic, which suggests it will likely persist. Working with our own anger will benefit not only us but everyone our life touches.

What causes this anger among healthcare professionals? I think there are several factors:

1. Opposing foundations: We base our lives and profession upon scientific information, research, evidence-based treatments, and reason. It is difficult to work with patients whose basis for medical decisions is the opposite: crowd-sourcing, rumors, conspiracy theories, and emotion.

2. Overturned expectations: We entered the medical field expecting most of our patients to be grateful for our care. When they are not only not grateful but are angry, disrespectful, and question our motives, it is distressing to us.

3. Sacrifice: Our careers require sacrifice, working long and sometimes double shifts, often not having time to eat or pee and missing family events and holidays. When people have no inkling of our sacrifices, it is hard.

4. Fear: Anger can arise out of fear when we are risking our own lives, our family's lives, and other patients' lives to care for someone, especially someone who resents our care.

5. Violating codes: Becoming angry with a patient violates our own code of professional conduct. It can make us angry at ourselves.

6. Existential crisis: When you combine hard work and sacrifices with disrespect and anger flung at you, you begin to wonder if this is the career for you. It can precipitate an existential crisis.

7. Moral injury: The COVID-19 pandemic heightened awareness of the moral crisis in medicine. Overwhelmed healthcare workers who had never been trained in making ethically complex and emotionally fraught decisions had to decide who would receive or be denied the care they needed, given shortages in staffing, space, and sup-

plies. Looked at more deeply, there is an inherent injustice in a healthcare system that does not provide good medical (and dental and mental health) care to everyone. How can people pursue life, liberty, and happiness in a country that denies them good health?

8. The sanctity of healthcare workers: There is evidence that the phenomenon of attacks on healthcare workers predated the pandemic. Before the pandemic, two nurses who work in an ER in a public hospital in San Francisco came to a Mindful Medicine retreat because of the stress of being physically assaulted by angry patients several times a month. Thirty percent of five thousand nurses surveyed in March 2021 said violence in the workplace was increasing. Some hospitals are giving panic buttons to their staff to summon security when they are attacked. One hospital administrator said, "When we were recruiting nursing students, it used to be that they would ask, 'How much money am I going to get paid? What department am I going to work in?' In 2018, nurses started asking, 'How are you going to protect me?'"[44]

9. Violating codes of conduct among healthcare workers: It is an unwritten law in healthcare that you do not make things more difficult for your fellow workers. You do not leave the next shift to cope with an IV that "just" came out or a patient with a full diaper or wound dressing that needed changing hours ago. Now burned-out healthcare workers are (understandably) quitting, leaving their friends even more overloaded. And hospitals are hiring traveling nurses who make three times the salary of the nurses who stayed on.

10. The fomented political divide in the nation: We never knew or cared before how our patients voted or what their religious beliefs were; we just took care of a sick human being. And patients didn't know how their doctors or nurses voted or prayed, either.

11. The corporate takeover of medicine: Most of us entered medicine as a career so we could help end, or at least mitigate, people's suffering, and we are now appalled to be chastised by administrators for not meeting patient "quotas" or for not capturing "our share of the patient load" in some specialty or department.

HOW TO WORK WITH ANGER

When we look deeply at the roots of our anger, we often discover that underneath anger is fear. For example, we are angry because we are afraid that injustices will never end, that new regimes will worsen the injustices in our or other countries. We may be afraid that injustices will invade our home.

Investigate this idea for yourself. Ask, "What am I worried might be the worst thing that could happen if this situation that makes me angry continues? And if that happens, what would be the worst thing that could happen as a result?" Keep digging.

For example, let's say you were quite angry at a patient who was angry at you. If this continues, "I might lose my job or quit." Then what is the very worst thing that could happen? "I wouldn't be able to find another job." And then? "I wouldn't be able to support myself or my family." "I would lose my status in the community and my coworkers and friends." And then? "I'd lose my house and be homeless. My spouse would leave me and my children would be ashamed of me. I wouldn't be able to feed myself." And then? "I'd die, hungry and alone, under a bridge." This conclusion might seem like a stretch, but our mind can be a "disaster-mongerer" as a Scottish friend once said. When it is afraid, in its attempt to protect us, our mind can go from A to Z, from angry patient to our lonely death, in an instant.

Finding and naming the fear underlying anger can be a relief and very helpful. Sometimes, we find that sadness is underneath anger. But isn't sadness actually a kind of fear—fear of loss? Loss of what we value: a person we love, money, possessions, status? Besides tracking the anger back to the fear that underlies it, there are a variety of ways to work with anger. Here are some suggestions:

- Use the Rescue Remedies from chapter 7 to bring your mind back into the present moment and away from perseverating on what happened. When we are angry, our focus narrows and our minds don't have perspective. You can go back to the incident of anger when your mind is clearer.
- Sleep on it. If you can, get some rest. Healthcare workers can be chronically tired, which is a risk factor for creating unhelpful reactions to stress.
- Understand that the person who provoked you or got angry with you is also afraid. When you are calm, ponder what it is that frightens them. It is not you, but something deeper. Wish loving kindness for them: may they be free from anger, may they be at ease, and may they find true happiness. And do it for yourself.
- Discern: will this problem be solved by me generating more anger? Or will anger only exacerbate the problem?

- Summon the three mindful self-compassion practices.
  Mindfulness: "I'm angry. This is difficult and doesn't feel good."

  Common humanity: "This is part of being human. Everyone feels anger at times in their lives, and many people around the world feel this way right now. I wish them and myself ease."

  Loving touch: Touch your hand, arm, or shoulder in a kind way, as a good friend would, and say, "I'm always here for you."
- Do something you love doing and fill your mind with that activity. Pay attention to your body. What are your hands feeling now? And now? Tell your mind that it needs to let go and rest for a while and that later it will be in better shape to look at what happened. Offer prayers or positive thoughts.
- Apologize. Apologizing is a hard, but necessary practice. It prevents the chain of anger from continuing and infecting others.

Some people worry about covering up their true feelings by substituting something else to occupy their mind. We are not covering anger up—we are acknowledging it and clearing space in our heart-mind so we can uncover its source and helpful insights can arise. Often finding its source will defuse or release the anger.

FINAL WORDS

Anger is the messenger, not the means to solve a problem. Seek its source. Convert its energy into clarity and determination.

Clearing Out the Day

THE PRACTICE

Each night before you get into bed, sit for a few moments (even on the edge of the bed) to review the day in your mind. You can do this every day for a week, or every evening for a month, but especially after any day that seemed difficult. There is an audio recording of this meditation that can help guide you through this exercise until you are easily able to do it by yourself (see www.shambhala.com/mindfulmedresources).

Play the day in your mind like a video being played in fast-forward, noticing things that pop out or stop the flow of the review. Begin with the time you arose, touching in on the things that you did today. For example, taking a shower, getting dressed, eating breakfast, driving to work, patients who might stick in your mind, attending meetings or grand rounds, eating lunch, telephone calls, meetings, driving home, what you did after you got home. Notice any events that stick out and catch your attention momentarily, then let them recede and join the stream of memories of the day.

If there are any reminder notes for tomorrow, write them now. Then consciously release. You can imagine the entire day dissolving or floating away in a helium balloon. The day that passed is just a dream. Let it go. It is gone and cannot be changed.

Some people prefer to let the fast video of the day flow backward; you can try it both ways and see which works best for you.

REMINDING YOURSELF

Put a note on your pillow that says, "Clear out the day."

DISCOVERIES

This practice is another favorite in our Mindful Medicine group.

It is an exercise I developed when I was seeing children who had been abused. Because children speak so frankly and often vividly about what happened to them, unpleasant images would stick in my mind. Sometimes, I would come home frustrated, feeling that I hadn't accomplished anything useful that day. In order to be able to sleep and then be fresh for the next day, I began doing this "video review." It helped free me of everything I had seen or heard and to release it into other hands.

Many doctors have asked me how to be able to let go of the human suffering they encounter each day. This is the best way I have found.

After you finish the review, you can say a small prayer along the lines of the loving kindness metta practice. "May I be free from anxiety, healthy, and at ease. May my patients be free from anxiety, healthy, and at ease." You can tailor this sincere wish to your own situation or needs, and add any individual, family member, coworker, or friend who arises in your mind.

Healthcare professionals say this exercise often surprises them. Instead of witnessing an apparently futile day of frustration and failure, they see that they were quite busy, worked diligently with every situation that arose, and gave their best. As one rural doctor said, "I see patients back-to-back all day, but when I do the fast-forward review, a few patients pop out. It gives the day more texture and helps me realize its depth." A number of doctors say it helps them let go of rumination and self-doubt and enter sleep in a more positive and relaxed state.

DEEPER LESSONS

So much of our energy is frittered away in ruminating about the past and in anxiety about the future. Our Inner Critic likes to bring up our past mistakes over and over, out of its terror that we will make another mistake in the future.

In the midst of a busy day, being pulled in multiple directions at once, barely finishing one task before running to the next, and a growing list of to-do items, we can lose perspective. It can seem as if we have accomplished nothing. When the negative predictions and judgments of the Inner Critic fill our mind, there's no room for remembering the many things we did competently and compassionately each day. A fast-forward or fast-backward video review of the day helps expand our awareness of the larger context, our daily life of service for others' benefit and healing.

Several people talked about waking up in the middle of the night when a pressing worry erupts into consciousness. In that half-awake state, we are quite vulnerable and unable to summon our usual problem-solving capacities. One doctor said she has a rule for her mind. "We will not think about this until after I get my coffee and the sun is out." She then imagines putting the problem on a very high shelf and going back to sleep. She says invoking this rule has taken determined practice, but is now easy to do.

It also helps us to recall that we are not in charge of the hundreds of thousands of actions of cause and effect that impinge daily upon our patients. We can only do our best in the small arena in which we play a transitory, walk-on-and-off, role.

FINAL WORDS

Refresh your heart and mind with a quick, dispassionate review of the day, release the day, and sleep well.

5

CONNECTING WITH YOUR PATIENTS

Why undertake mindfulness practices to help you connect with your patients? Simple. Connecting more effectively with patients can support two things many of us hoped for in taking on a career in healthcare: helping people to heal and providing the satisfaction of knowing we have lived a meaningful life. It can also help us avoid three things that cause us medical people anxiety: mistakes that harm patients, negative reviews on social media, and lawsuits.

Humans are social animals; we thrive in an atmosphere of kindness and gratitude. Research shows that the voice, the touch, or even the silent presence of a caring partner can mitigate pain.[1]

Unfortunately, the productivity demands of corporate medicine dictate shorter patient visits and thus less time to settle in with a person and weave strands of connection and trust. Doctors who are in the throes of burning out find themselves seeing patients as just a diagnosis—"I can't see another diabetic with out-of-control eating today!"—or becoming irritated and short with patients—"If you can't follow my recommendations, I'm not interested in seeing you again."

EMPATHY

You already have empathy and compassion, or you wouldn't be working in healthcare.[2] There was a time when some people became physicians because of the prestige or money involved in that career. Now the burden of paying off the cost of college and medical school can last for years. Add in the expense of malpractice insurance and the monetary incentive evaporates. Although nurses have become more empowered, earn decent salaries, and have been ranked the most trusted, ethical, and honest profession for nineteen years in a row, they face increased stress and high rates of burnout.[3] Doctors used to be honored pillars of the community. Now patients have less trust in the medical system and may challenge their doctor with a self-made diagnosis and demands for treatment they have read about on the web. We ponder prescribing a "googlectomy."

What keeps us in our jobs when honor and riches evaporate? We care. We are moved by the pain of other human beings and we want to help relieve their suffering.

Our professions require a balance between empathy and detachment, between openheartedness and clear-mindedness. We can't collapse with grief as a badly injured accident victim is wheeled in the ER nor can we be indifferent and cold as we inform their waiting family of their loved person's true condition. However, our caring, open hearts are not a one-way street. Over the months and years in the fray, bit by bit, the sorrow of the human condition seeps in and our hearts gradually fill up. Our daily witnessing of this sorrow begins to overwhelm our daily experience of its beauty, even majesty. To protect our own hearts, we can tip over into emotional detachment and need help in recovering our natural ability to feel emotional attunement.

Empathy has amazing power. Research has documented the many benefits of empathic listening on patient outcomes: increased immune function, shorter post-surgery hospital stays, shorter healing times (even from a common cold), better levels of hemoglobin A1c in diabetics, decreased asthma attacks, and better psychological adjustment to illness.[4] From a patient's perspective, their doctor or nurse is empathic if they express compassion and concern for the patient's well-being and seem to understand how a patient feels and thinks. Patients who perceive physicians as more empathic have increased trust, will disclose more information about their condition, and show better compliance with treatment. Patients who rate their physicians as more empathic also rate themselves as more satisfied with their care.[5]

Empathy can be (re)learned. Because of this compelling research, training in empathy has been added to the curriculum in many medical schools. Besides reopening a shuttered heart, there are other important benefits for a healthcare provider. Doctors who communicate well and show empathy with their patients are less likely to be sued and have lower rates of burnout.[6]

The mindfulness practices in this chapter are designed with attention to the clues patients actually use to decide whether a physician is connecting with them and showing empathy: eye contact, active listening, kind touch, and interest in the patient's life outside of the medical encounter.

HEALTHCARE PROVIDER, HEAL THYSELF

In a way, the division between mindfulness practices that helps you connect with yourself and those that help you connect with your patients is an artificial division. All of the exercises in this chapter on connecting with your patients apply to you. If you do what you prescribe, have your own hobby, a pet, or plants, if you investigate your own worries and fears, gather sources of support for yourself, and keep your mind open to what is working (rather than obsessing about what is not), you will be healing yourself as well.

Some of the exercises in chapter 4, like Breathing Together and Loving Hands, Healing Touch will also expand your awareness of your patients' bodies, hearts, and minds. Medicine is not a one-way outward energetic flow. If we practice it in that way, we will go down in flames. Mindfulness helps us nourish and care for ourselves at the same time we nourish and care for our patients.

Talking about What Is Working Well

When speaking to patients, intentionally talk about the parts of the body that are working well before you focus on the problem organs or areas. This idea can apply when talking about mental or emotional health and well-being as well.

For example, when going over labs, instead of immediately saying, "Your lab work is normal except for . . ." you might say something like this: "Your lab work shows that your kidneys are working quite well, maintaining the balance of salts, nitrogen, proteins, and water in your body. And according to the blood work, your liver is also in good shape. Your white blood cells, which can help fight infection, and your red blood cells, which carry oxygen from your lungs to your cells, are all circulating in good numbers. It looks like you might need some supplemental iron to support your red blood cells."

Or "Your blood sugar is normal, which means that your pancreas is doing a good job monitoring changes in your blood sugar and secreting appropriate amounts of insulin. You can support your pancreas by minimizing the amount of processed food and sugar that you eat." This approach is in line with research showing that if you need to deliver a negative message and want to optimize how it is received, it should be "sandwiched" between positive messages.

While doing the physical exam, you might say, "Your lungs and heart sound good, and your blood pressure is fine. Your surgical incision is healing well. Isn't it amazing how so many parts of your body are functioning so well by themselves?"

REMINDING YOURSELF

Put a note: "What is working!" on your computer where you'll see it as you check old or new lab results.

DISCOVERIES

This exercise brought delight to the healthcare professionals in our Mindful Medicine group. One physician who tried this practice called it "ingenious," in taking the focus of the provider and the patient off "the problem" while still communicating important messages. It can be helpful with teens, who are bombarded by enhanced, filtered images of perfect bodies, faces, and hair on social media and worry about small imperfections that are inconsequential to the doctor, like asymmetry of their labia.[7]

It doesn't just apply to physical findings or lab values. Another physician, on the first day at a new administrative job, found her anxiety growing as things began going wrong. She switched her mental focus to "what is working well" and found her mood and enthusiasm for the job lifted immediately. A family practice doctor mentioned applying this practice to psychological issues such as tension and conflict between teens and parents. He tried asking first, "Tell me what's working."

In medical interactions, we often focus on the problem areas, what part or parts of the body are not working optimally. We look over a lab report and our eyes slide past all the normal values and fixate on the abnormal values. Now that our patients have access to their medical record, they do the same, but they don't have enough medical training to know that an "abnormal value" may be only a tiny fraction outside the normal range or that normal values can vary with age. So they worry needlessly.

I had a friend who had a PET scan as a way to check how his chemotherapy was progressing. Aspects of the radiologist's report that he had no framework for made him quite anxious for several days until he could talk to his doctor, who reassured him that these were incidental findings and not a sign that the cancer was returning. And if he had gone on the web to try to interpret the radiologist's report, it would have made things worse.

I've had three inspirations for this practice of speaking about what works. Ten months after a partial knee replacement, I went to see the surgeon to complain about the clicking sounds in my knee. He looked at me as I sat cross-legged on the exam table, palpated and manipulated my leg, commented on my good muscle strength, and then said, "Your outcome far surpasses what we expect from this surgery. You are a superstar!" In an instant, I went from feeling that I was defective to feeling like a superstar. Whenever I get discouraged about how age limits what I can do, I hear him call me "superstar" and my spirits instantly lift.

The second inspiration was a video by Jon Kabat-Zinn. Years ago, some hospitals played this video on their in-house television channels for pre-operative and post-operative patients. Doctors on rounds could "prescribe" that their patients "take" this mindfulness exercise twice or three times a day as a way to actively participate in their healing. In the video (which is still available), Kabat-Zinn gently guided people to move into the full experience of the present moment and their current circumstances.[8] He also had patients focus on everything in their body that was working perfectly, day and night, to care for them—and there was just one part that needed some help. This inspired me to develop the Gratitude for the Body meditation, which appears in chapter 6.

My third inspiration has been what seems to be a new trend in dentistry: patient-centered care. Instead of scolding me for how long it had been since my last cleaning or for what I was doing wrong, my dentist began emphasizing the positive. When my dentist asked how often I flossed, and I truthfully answered, "Once a week," my dentist said, "Oh, that's great, but it really works best if you do it once a day. I'm noticing a fair amount of plaque and that's where the bacteria lurk that cause cavities. I have some new dental flossers you might like better than string floss. Give them a try." No one particularly looks forward to dental visits and being chastised doesn't help.

As one dentist observes, "As children, many of us were taught the Golden Rule—treat others as you want to be treated. A patient-centered care approach for dentistry . . . demands that we instead adopt the Platinum Rule—treat others as they want to be treated. . . . There is no script to follow that relates to all of our patients. Each patient presents with unique needs and demands that need to be identified, respected and addressed."[9]

DEEPER LESSONS

One of my mottos is, "The mind is magnetically attracted to the negative." This is proved by the news. If you count how many stories in the news lineup are negative, it's usually 90 percent or more. There's often one feel-good story about a dog that jumped out of a car and found its way home through a snowstorm or a kid who started a charity to recycle contact lenses.[10]

Our mind wants to keep us safe, so it is extra alert to dangers—and the world is full of them. The news pours the woes of the world into our eyes, minds, and hearts every day. Our body and heart-mind evolved over 200,000 years to take in the suffering of a small tribe or village, not the entire world. Just as our mind slides past the normal values and fixates on the abnormal, our mind slides over the myriad things in our life—or in the world—that are going well and gnaws on what it perceives as a problem. To be able to cope with the onslaught of information about unending tragedies and dangers, we need a reliable antidote. I have found mindfulness and meditation to be the best medicine for this persistent feeling of dis-ease, anxiety about the condition of our earth, and the beings who live in and on it.

The promise of mindfulness is that when we recognize a state of mind or heart that is difficult or harmful, we can change it. It takes practice. We've practiced letting our mind follow the same path—actual neural pathways—to the old, familiar comfort of anxiety for decades. It will take sustained practice to notice where our mind is headed, then pick it up, and shift it to mindfulness; that is, full attention to what is actually happening right now, the feeling of the earth supporting us under our feet, the warm breath leaving our nostrils, or what our fingertips are touching. You can try it right now. Just stop thinking and put your awareness in your amazing body.

Practicing gratitude, becoming aware of all that is working well, helps us make the shift to appreciating what is always supporting us, unnoticed in the background, what we take for granted. We can help our patients make this shift too when we emphasize what is working well in their bodies and their lives.

FINAL WORDS

Nothing thrives under negative attention. Not children, animals, or even plants. Our body and our patient's bodies are no exception.

Asking about Hobbies—
And Undertaking a Hobby

THE PRACTICE

Ask at least one or two patients each week about their hobbies. You can directly ask, "Do you have any hobbies?" If they don't understand or say they don't have hobbies, you can ask, "Do you do any crafts, like sewing, knitting, or wood carving . . . or do you play any instruments, or sing . . . or dance or do yoga . . . or cook for fun? Do you collect anything?" If they still say they have no hobbies, you can ask, "What do you enjoy doing in your free time?"

Another way to begin this conversation is to provide a Hobby Information Sheet for patients to fill out in the waiting room. An example is at the link in the notes.[11]

If you discover a hobby, ask a few follow-up questions about how they got started in their hobby or why they enjoy doing it. Make a note of their hobbies in their medical record for future reference.

DISCOVERIES

Patients are often surprised, and then pleased, when a doctor asks about a positive aspect of their personal life. It signals that they aren't just an anonymous body, but a unique, interesting human being. Remember that a primary fear of patients is depersonalization. And a primary human need is connection.

You may be surprised, too. Finding out about a patient's hobbies can give you clues about their health, for example, such as working with potentially hazardous substances like dry clay, paint fumes, or wood dust. You might discover a mutual hobby or a dangerous activity such as BASE jumping. One physician discovered that she and her patient were both painters and talked about good sources for supplies. Asking about hobbies can lend depth to your interaction and form the basis for continued conversation at their next visit. Returning patients are often happy that you remembered their hobbies or special interests.

When you read the abundant research on the benefits of hobbies on physical and mental health, you realize that we should be prescribing hobbies for our patients, and for ourselves.

Engaging in an enjoyable hobby has been correlated with lower blood pressure, smaller waist circumference, lower levels of depression, and higher levels of positive psychosocial states.[12] An extensive literature review and original study of more than two thousand people, part of the Midlife Development in the United States (MIDUS) study, indicated that daily stressors (such as meeting work deadlines, traffic jams, or arguments with someone close to you) have a stronger impact on health than chronic stressors (including chronic health issues). Leisure-time activities, plus "leisure-time sufficiency," can facilitate recovery from daily stressors.[13]

If you want to find a new job, an article from a "physician head-hunter" company recommends hiring physicians who have hobbies because research shows that hobbies can "enhance leadership skills and make doctors more resilient during stressful situations."[14] People who have engaging hobbies are better able to transition from work overload to time-on-their-hands during retirement. A charming article from the *Journal of the American Medical Association* one hundred years ago extols the importance of hobbies for physicians, for just this reason.[15] A recent survey of how physicians spend their time outside of the exam room found that about half enjoy reading and gourmet cooking in their leisure time and about a third like to walk, run, bicycle, or attend cultural or arts events.[16] Some physicians take on unusual hobbies such as stand-up comedy.[17]

A study of nephrology nurses showed that burnout was significantly higher in those who did not have a hobby. One hobby was enough, and it did not matter if the hobby involved physical activity or not.[18] Advocating hobbies for healthcare personnel, an orthopedic surgeon wrote, "The point is any singular activity that rests your nervous system and diverts attention from the continual vigilance that a medical vocation demands will add years and joy to one's life."

DEEPER LESSONS

Hobbies can be a connection to something bigger than ourselves. One of my practices is to try to find in someone's hobby an underlying connection to what we might call the Divine or the Greater Mystery within our ordinary life. For example, work with clay reflects creation stories about humans being created from clay. An underlying lesson of these stories is that just as all colors of clay are beautiful to the potter, so all colors of skin are beautiful to the creator. Many hobbies involve creation and support our desire to add the warmth of love to a handmade gift or to leave something of value behind when we die.

Reflect for a moment on the calcium in your body. How old is it? When was it created?

The answer is billions of years old, created by explosions of massive or white dwarf stars. How many living organisms has that calcium passed through before it became part of your teeth and bones? Billions. And when you die and return that calcium to the earth, how many bodies will it pass through in the future? Billions. We are like clay pots, continually created on a great potter's wheel, serving a purpose, destroyed, and shaped again into a different form.

When people become immersed in their hobbies, they often lose track of time. As mentioned earlier in the discussion of "flow," certain activities help us release the emergency brake of the mind's anxieties—which makes it let go of its constant detours into past and future—and allow us to enter the stream of the ceaseless, effortless flow of this moment, this moment, this moment. This is a territory of respite and relaxation, outside of our overcrowded calendar and personal worries.

The Inner Critic has no traction in the present moment. That is why activities that immerse us in the present moment make us feel refreshed and happy.

FINAL WORDS

Do you have a hobby? Do you meditate or sit in silence in contemplative prayer? Do you have other ways to rest in the present moment and be refreshed? These are ways we can heal ourselves.

Noticing Eye Color

THE PRACTICE

Notice your patients' eye color. Note: This involves directly looking at them while talking to them. Record their eye color in their chart. In addition to blue or brown, notice different shades of gray, green, or gold. At the same time, you could take note of any vertical earlobe creases.[19]

REMINDING YOURSELF

Put a sticky note on your computer screen or someplace obvious in your office saying, "Eye Color."

DISCOVERIES

We medical professionals are often in a hurry, preoccupied with the busyness of getting through a patient visit and on to the next. We look at the computer as we enter data in the e-chart or as we scribble notes, asking patients questions as we continue to type or write.

It is impossible to pay full attention to two things at once. Prove this yourself with a simple experiment. Close your eyes and bring full awareness to your right big toe. Notice all the sensations that tell you that you have a big toe: temperature, tingling, touch, pressure. Now move your full attention to your left earlobe. Since you cannot see it, how do you know you have an earlobe? Be aware of all the sensations: temperature, tingling, touch, pressure.

Now pay full attention to both your right big toe and your left earlobe. What do you notice? Can you pay full attention to both?

Or is your attention weakened, divided, or fluctuating, flitting back and forth?

We have to acknowledge that we cannot pay full attention to a patient while entering data into a computer. We've all had conversations with someone who was distracted, who was cracking their knuckles or neck or moving their eyes away to look over our shoulder. It's frustrating, especially if the conversation is important to you, like a conversation about your worrisome physical symptoms or upcoming surgery. A review of literature on bedside manner found that relationship-focused training, which included maintaining eye contact, had a small but statistically significant effect on the specific health outcomes in patients with obesity, diabetes, asthma, or osteoarthritis. It could affect weight loss, blood pressure, blood sugar, lipid levels, and pain. Interestingly, the researchers noted that the impact was greater than the reported effects of low-dose aspirin or cholesterol-lowering statins for preventing heart attack.[20]

What do we know about eye color? Eye color is determined by a number of genes, not a single gene as we might have learned in biology classes. Any combination of parent-child eye color is possible. There is no blue or green pigment in blue or green eyes; those colors are due to light scattering, similar to the cause of the apparent blue color of the sky.

Eye color ranges from light blue to dark brown. Scientists believe that originally all humans had brown eyes; blue eyes may be the result of one mutation that occurred only six to ten thousand years ago. Blue eyes are found in just 8–10 percent of people in the world and are becoming less common. Eye color is also related to a higher risk of having a number of diseases. Blue-eyed people have a higher risk of type 1 diabetes, hearing loss, melanoma, infiltrating endotheliosis, and age-related macular degeneration, but have higher pain tolerance in labor.[21] Brown-eyed people are more likely to develop vitiligo and cataracts.[22] One study found that blue-eyed people are more likely to drink alcohol, drink larger amounts, and have a higher risk of developing alcoholism.[23] Heterochromia, two different eye colors in the same person, can be a familial trait, or the result of chimerism—having two complete sets of DNA. If heterochromia appears late in life, it can be a sign of disease such as pigmented glaucoma or neurofibromatosis. If you notice heterochromia in an infant or if one eye changes color later in life, a medical workup and a referral to an ophthalmologist are warranted.

You might comment on positive aspects of this research to a patient, saying something like, "I notice you have blue eyes. Did you know that blue-eyed people are less susceptible to cataracts?" Or, for a brown-eyed person, "Did you know that brown-eyed people seem to be less likely to get into trouble with alcohol?" We can educate people in informal as well as formal ways.

DEEPER LESSONS

We look at rashes and moles, in ears and down throats, at nail beds and clubbing, we check mouths for tongue cancer and dental caries, and we might use the ophthalmoscope to check for pupillary reflexes and papilledema, but we don't often look patients directly in the eye, human being to human being.

Many of our patients live relatively lonely lives. Our connection with them might be the only warm interaction of their day. Research shows that when physicians make eye contact with patients during a visit, patients rate the physician as more empathic and are more satisfied with their care. The effect of eye contact will increase the patient's empathy rating for the doctor even when the length of the visit is short.[24]

Making eye contact in healthcare is not without complexity; looking into another person's eyes may make us uncomfortable because it seems too intimate. Women may develop a tendency to watch people's mouths as they talk, rather than look into their eyes. This is a protective habit, formed to prevent men from misinterpreting direct gaze as an invitation. There are cultural differences, too. In some cultures, particularly Muslim or Asian, women are often taught not to have direct eye contact with men. In other cultures, maintaining eye contact can be seen as a sign of self-confidence. Direct eye contact can confer feelings of honesty and sincerity, but prolonged eye contact may be seen as exerting power or sexual interest. However, in Asian, African, Native American, or Latin American cultures prolonged direct eye contact can signal disrespect or even anger.[25]

Healthcare providers may be hesitant to look directly into the eyes of their patients, for fear of misinterpretation of those actions as sexual interest or concern about triggering reactions related to past trauma. This is an area where we need to be sensitive, but not tip over into being cold and overly formal.

I've found that I learn a lot about how to behave as a physician when I am on the other side—as a patient. My primary care physician always sits at my level and looks me in the eye as we begin conversing at the start of the visit, and it makes me feel more connected, more trusting, and open to telling her all my concerns. It's a small difference, but one I notice every time I see her. Her warm but gentle handshake at the beginning or end of our visit is also quite effective.

FINAL WORDS

When we are busy, it's all too easy to begin objectifying patients. And, by association, ourselves. A few moments of connecting, by looking into their eyes as you greet them and asking about their concerns, can make a big difference to both of you.

Asking about Pets or Plants

THE PRACTICE

Ask patients if they have a pet.

If they do, ask a bit more about the pet's name, breed or color, age, temperament, and what they like best about the pet. Remember that birds, aquarium fish, and reptiles can be pets. If they don't have a personal pet, ask about whether they have frequent contact with animals or if they have houseplants or garden plants that they tend.

REMINDING YOURSELF

Put a small note that says "PETS or PLANTS" on your computer screen or clipboard, where you will notice it as you check or make entries in the patient's medical record.

DISCOVERIES

This is a practice the healthcare providers in our Mindful Medicine group always enjoy. Those who have tried asking about pets say that it creates an immediate connection; an anxious or taciturn patient will visibly brighten up and begin to happily chat about their pet. It's a good way to engage with a shy child or cautious teenager.

There is voluminous literature on the many benefits of having a pet or even having access to a pet. The benefits are so clear, it seems odd that medical and mental healthcare workers do not routinely ask about pets. The CDC and the NIH have summarized the health benefits of owning and caring for a pet to include: lower blood pressure, increased exercise, better fitness, reduced levels of depression and anxiety, and lower levels of cholesterol, triglycerides, and cortisol. A growing body of research documents the benefits of pets to children with attention problems, hyperactivity, and autism.[26] A study of over one million children in Sweden showed that growing up with a dog or on a farm during the first six years of life significantly reduced the chances that a child would develop asthma. It seems that exposure to certain types and amounts of animal-associated microbes early in life helps us develop a healthy immune system.[27]

Over 60 percent of homes in the United States include a pet, and 95 percent of pet owners consider their pet to be a family member.[28] Children often confide their feelings to a pet and feel that the pet understands and loves them just as they are. For older patients, especially as their children leave home and/or their spouse dies, their pets become their children and companions.

People who cannot own a pet can benefit from sessions of pet therapy. Pet therapy sessions in nursing homes have been shown to reduce depression, anxiety, apathy, agitation, and feelings of loneliness and increase cognitive skills and the quality of life for elderly people residing there.[29] Just thirty minutes a day observing aquarium fish increased mental function, alertness, memory, verbalization, and food intake in patients with Alzheimer's.[30]

Talking to a patient about their pets is not irrelevant to your medical assessment. You may notice that a patient becomes more animated when talking about their pets. Or, if a pet is ill or has recently died, you may see signs of grief, anxiety, or depression. You might ask how the pet helps its owner.

Ask about how many cats, dogs, or birds they have. You could discover a home overrun with dozens of stray cats. I had a friend whose two little finches—male and female—morphed into a large smelly living room filled with dozens of cages with feathers and crunchy birdseed on the floor. She couldn't bear to discard any of the eggs they laid.

You might discover dangerous pets. Babies and children have been killed by family pets such as aggressive dogs and wild animals such as ferrets, boa constrictors, pythons, chimpanzees, and big cats. Horses can be pets, as can other farm animals.

Remember that 40 percent of homes in the United States don't include pets. If your patient does not have a pet, be sure to ask about plants they care for. A psychiatric nurse practitioner in our Mindful Medicine group was so impressed with the evidence that plants enhance the physical and mental health of patients and staff that he immediately bought five plants for his office.

Asking about a pet or plants may open up new areas of conversation and connection. Asking about something outside the routine medical questions shows that you care not just about the disease but about the whole, unique person, one who has come to you in a vulnerable position.

DEEPER LESSONS

In Maslow's hierarchy of needs, after physiological needs (food, drink, warmth, shelter) and safety needs are met, the next higher level of basic human need is for love and intimacy, trust, a feeling of belonging, and the ability to give and receive affection.

A meta-analysis and review of research on the effect on the mental well-being of people living with a mental illness of having pets (including cats, dogs, hamsters, finches, and goldfish) found that pets helped patients manage their emotions and distracted them from the symptoms of their mental illness.[31] The study includes touching narratives from clients. They said that pets gave them unconditional acceptance and love, which they were often not receiving from their family or other people. They commented that the pet could intuitively sense when the owner was distressed and moved closer to give them comfort and a sense of calm. They described being able to confide in their pets without fear of being interrupted, judged, criticized, or their confidence being betrayed.

Taking care of an animal gave these patients a sense of purpose, meaning, and self-worth in their lives, and even prevented suicide, as they did not want to abandon the animal. Walking a pet helped them take physical exercise and stay in touch with their neighbors—whom they met on walks—and with their community. Those with pets were also more likely to use ambulatory healthcare services.

The authors of the review article called for a cultural change that promotes the therapeutic benefits of pets for people with mental health issues. Wouldn't we all benefit from a companion who is a nonjudgmental listener and provides unconditional affection and physical warmth? Or one who distracts us from our mental distress and often injects humor into our life?

If a patient does not have a pet, ask about whether they have houseplants or do gardening. There is extensive literature on the benefit of plants showing that caring for a plant can enhance mental and physical health.[32] For example, one group of residents in a nursing home was given choices about how they could arrange their furniture, were allowed to move about where and when they wanted, could spend time with whom they wanted, and were given the option of accepting a plant to care for. The control group was told that the staff was there to take care of them, including watering a plant given to each of them. Though only marginally significant, results indicated that during this study period and eighteen months later, residents in the group that were given increased control over their environment and direct care of a plant had improved health and none had died. Several patients in the group who were not given choices or care for another living being had died.[33]

Simply looking at plants induces subjective and objective measures of relaxation, as we saw in the Nature Bathing practice. Surgical patients in one study who had living plants in their hospital rooms had significantly lower systolic blood pressure and lower ratings of pain, anxiety, and fatigue than patients in the control rooms without plants. Patients' comments indicated that plants in their room gave them the positive impression that hospital employees cared about their patients.[34]

Horticultural (gardening) therapy has been shown to reduce stress and depression, increase overall happiness and life satisfaction, reduce symptoms of trauma and speed recovery of people who are traumatized by natural disasters, and mitigate PTSD in veterans and ADHD.[35]

We humans evolved in an environment replete with animals and plants of every kind. Look around your office to see if it is devoid of plants. Consider an aquarium in your waiting room or a trained therapy dog if you do counseling. If you spend a few hours reading the research on the benefits of pets and plants, you may end up with a jungle for an office and a zoo at home!

FINAL WORDS

Pets and plants are effective medicine, for you and for those you care for.

Absorptive Compassionate Listening

THE PRACTICE

When you are listening to a patient, allow your mind to become quiet and fully attentive to what you are hearing. We sometimes call this "listen like a sponge," soaking up what the other person is saying.

Don't formulate a response until it is requested or obviously needed.

REMINDING YOURSELF

Post the words, "Listen like a sponge" or a drawing or picture of an ear or a sponge on the computer you use during the patient visit or on the hand sanitizer or soap dispenser where you wash your hands before you talk with your patients.

DISCOVERIES

Attentive listening is not easy. We are used to mental multitasking, hearing both what the other person is saying and also what our own mind is saying—or wants to say—in response. We are listening while also worrying about the last patient or a problem at home or making a mental shopping list or wondering what is causing the loud noise in the hall outside. We may feel rushed and interrupt our patient, worrying that if we spend too much time listening to one patient, we will keep the next one waiting.

To listen with a completely quiet, alert mind is a very valuable skill. Experienced counselors often say that attentive, open-hearted listening is the most important therapeutic tool they have. They are alert to subtle changes in the tone or a catch in the voice that belies what the client is saying and can reveal hidden emotions.

Lawyers, on the other hand, are trained to be listening for the flaws in a witness' statements. As they listen, they are planning how they will rebut what is being said. "Rebuttal mind" may be a valuable skill in the courtroom, but it is not likely to be appreciated in conversations at home, especially with spouses or teenage children.

One hospitalist wrote about her experience trying to convince a claustrophobic patient to have an MRI. The doctor was getting nowhere; the patient was adamant in her refusal. The doctor said, "That's when it struck me. I talked. I explained. I educated. I reasoned. But I had forgotten one of the most important aspects of medicine. I had not taken the time to actually listen to my patient." When she asked the patient why she had severe claustrophobia, the patient told her about being locked in a small dark space for a long period of time in childhood and the mental health consequences that followed. After her doctor listened to her halting and emotional disclosure with compassion, the patient spontaneously agreed to the MRI.[36]

Active or absorptive listening includes the following:

- turning your body toward your patient and looking at their face
- listening like a sponge, with a quiet, open, and curious mind
- giving back a summary of what you heard: "I think I heard you say . . . "

- asking questions to clarify: "I need to ask a few questions to clarify what is happening. Does the pain wake you up at night?"
- listening for and asking about underlying fears or beliefs: "What about this worries you?"
- expressing empathy: "That must have been hard for you."

Research on malpractice suits showed that 71 percent were caused by a problem in the physician-patient relationship. The most litigious patients felt that their physician was uncaring. Poor listening by the physician was a reason for lawsuits in 13 percent of cases.[37] Patients who are dissatisfied now have the ability to leave negative feedback on the web, another incentive for us to learn and practice active listening.

If you watch your mind, you may find that while you are listening to a patient recount their symptoms, you are simultaneously running through a mental differential diagnosis and beginning to plan which diagnostic tests to order or medication to prescribe. If we don't listen carefully and don't ask questions to clarify vague symptoms, we may jump to conclusions that delay the correct diagnosis and treatment.[38]

DEEPER LESSONS

One expert in attentive listening, Julian Treasure, says that with the popularity of social media, we have shifted from listening to broadcasting. We broadcast videos of our breakfasts, our latest dance moves, makeup routines, pranks, TEDx Talks, epic fails, adorable pets/children, and beautifully decorated birthday cakes. The art of the give and take of thoughtful conversations is being lost under this barrage. He suggests training in mindful listening.[39]

Most people have not had the experience of being completely listened to. By itself, it can be therapeutic. One of our students who came from a home where no one was interested in what he had to say told us that having someone listen to him with undivided attention was like receiving "life-giving mana."

Moments of silence are a rare but vital element in conscious communication. One doctor who specializes in diabetes told me that when she doesn't know how to move forward with a patient who is having problems, she asks the patient to take a few minutes with her in silence to clear their minds and see if a solution might arise. She has been surprised at how often they, she and the patient together, are then able to come up with a workable strategy.

We are more likely to have the ability to drop into a clear, quiet, receptive mind if we have spent a significant time in meditation, especially a multi-day silent meditation retreat. We are more likely to utilize the option of an open, alert mind if we have experienced the unexpected insight that can arise from it. Not everyone has the opportunity for a multi-day retreat, but anyone can experience the inner peace that results from cultivating a quiet, open, listening mind.

Whenever I have a problem that is tangled up in my mind, I go out in the garden to weed. As much as possible, I let go of thinking and open my senses to the colors, shapes, and sounds around me, and to what my hands are experiencing. Often, after about thirty minutes, a new way of looking at or handling the situation spontaneously arises. It has happened so often that I have come to trust it. Letting go of thinking, opening up to what is, allows the answer to my dilemma to appear.

What activity do you have that helps you drop thinking and rest in awareness? This takes us back to the importance of hobbies for our mental and physical well-being. It could be golfing, knitting, painting, hiking, fishing, or just sitting and watching the flames in the fireplace. My pediatrician friend used to come home from his office, change clothes, and sit in an easy chair with earphones on, listening to classical music for twenty minutes. Then he was ready to be a husband and father. His family knew the benefit and respected his "reset" time.

FINAL WORDS

Remember to listen with a quiet mind.

And when you talk, converse with patients instead of talking at them.

Asking about Fears and Worries

THE PRACTICE

For one week, try asking patients about their biggest fear or worry about their health or current illness, or anything they are concerned about in their life. You may need to adjust how you ask the question for each patient and situation. "Do you have any worries about your health right now that it might help to tell me?" "What are the biggest challenges in your life right now?" A psychiatric nurse practitioner remarked that he wouldn't use the word *fear* with his patients with paranoia, but a gentler word, like *concerns*.

If you do this for a month, it could become a small research study. I was surprised to find that there is very little research on this topic. You could keep a simple tally of the results and discover the most common fears or anxieties in your patient population.

REMINDING YOURSELF

Post a small note "Fear or worry?" on the screen of the computer you use to access the electronic medical record.

DISCOVERIES

I discovered the importance of asking patients about their greatest fear when I was a resident. I was evaluating a boy about ten years old in the outpatient clinic who presented with headaches. He did not have auras, nausea, facial pain, tearing, facial flushing, or any other abnormal symptoms. He was not awakened by headaches at night and change of position did not exacerbate the pain. The headaches occurred after school, during the school week, not on the weekends, and were relieved by a short rest. His physical growth and exam were normal. He had no papilledema nor any neurological abnormalities.

I went through the differential diagnosis with his mother, saying that he did not have any signs of migraines or histamine headaches and that he seemed to have tension headaches. We talked about sources of stress, and I suggested counseling.

I could see that she was not satisfied with my explanation. I had purposely not mentioned brain tumor as I reviewed possible diagnoses with her, for three reasons: brain tumors are extremely rare in a young child, his history and physical exam gave no sign of increased intracranial pressure, and I did not want to implant the alarming possibility of a brain tumor if the mother had not thought of it already.

Because my words of reassurance were clearly having no effect, I asked her what her greatest fear was about these headaches. She blurted out, "I'm afraid it might be a brain tumor. His uncle has a brain tumor, and I'm afraid it might be catching." As she said this, the tension in the air dissolved. I was able to reassure her about the specific fear she carried, and she relaxed. It was a fear I considered almost absurd, but until it was acknowledged, we were getting nowhere.

I have carried this lesson with me through my medical career. When I worked evaluating children for abuse, I often encountered parents who were not the ones who had injured their child, but who were nonetheless resistant to answering my questions, even belligerent. I found that if I asked them, "What is your greatest fear about what might happen as a result of today's evaluation?" and they were able to tell me, things completely changed. Usually, their fear was that their children would be taken away from them. I was able to give them some reassurance that if they were able to follow our recommendations, their child would remain at home. Their resistance dropped, and we were able to continue with the evaluation.

Even when the diagnosis is a dire one, such as cancer, asking the question about the greatest fear can yield unexpected answers. Hair loss? Loss of sexual function? Disfigurement? Inability to bear pain? Abandonment by their partner? Dying? Leaving small children without a parent? Fear of what happens after death?

Just bringing the fear out in the open and naming it can be a relief. And it provides a chance for us to address that fear, or at least to reassure them that we will be with them, caring for and supporting them, no matter what happens.

The spectrum of emotions based in fear runs from nervousness through anxiety, dread, panic, and terror. Chronic fear or anxiety can trigger arousal of the sympathetic nervous system and release of adrenaline and cortisol. This is not a healthy long-term state for our patients or for us. I've noticed that screening questionnaires given out in doctors' waiting rooms ask about symptoms of depression or about recent falls, but not about fears, anxieties, or worries.

About one-third of adults in the United States have an anxiety disorder at some time in their life. (This increased to 40% during the COVID-19 pandemic.)[40] If we knew that one-third of our patients were going to get diabetes, we would surely screen for it. Surprisingly, one international study involving in-person mental health interviews with almost fifteen thousand people found that anxiety levels were much lower in low-income countries (1.6 percent) compared to high-income countries (5.0 percent). The authors speculate that "there may be greater demands on individuals in higher-income countries to achieve independence, occupational success, and social status in a competitive environment, increasing uncertainty and perceived pressure to meet high expectation" and that people who have more wealth and possessions may have more worry about losing them in the future.[41]

DEEPER LESSONS

Chronic anxiety and accompanying sympathetic arousal have consequences for the health of our body, including elevated blood pressure, irritable bowel syndrome, immune dysfunction, and coronary artery disease.[42] In my experience, fear, and its somewhat milder cousin, anxiety, are the most pervasive destroyers of happiness in modern society. Chronic anxiety can be insidious; many people don't recognize it in themselves. When I've asked people what would happen if they weren't anxious, they have said, "I'd fail," or "I'd be too comfortable and I wouldn't get out of bed in the morning." One person pondered and then said, "I'd be average."

I love this answer, although it is sad, too. To be average is a form of failure in a culture that gives the prizes to the person who clambers over their friends and coworkers and finally stands on top of the heap with a gold medal around their neck. In other cultures, group harmony, cooperation, and group success are more highly valued than individual success.

Doctors are generally better at caring for patients' physical concerns rather than their emotional needs. We often leave that to the nurses, social workers, or therapists who have training in this important aspect of therapeutic skill. One physician in our Mindful Medicine group says she starts each visit by asking, "We know that stress affects our health. Can you tell me how things are going for you . . . in your life . . . with your family . . . with your work . . . and with your health?" This seems like a bold thing to do, as it invites patients to talk about many aspects of their life, but she has learned that it actually saves her time. For example, if she doesn't start by announcing that the patient's lab work shows an A1c level of 12 (an indication of high blood sugars over the past three months) and describing how they will tackle this, through her initial questions she can discover that the patient's mother died a week ago, the patient just flew back on a red-eye from the funeral, and the adult children are fighting over the will. She said, "Now I know why the A1c is elevated, and we can address the real issues: grief and stress."

Healthcare providers might be apprehensive about asking about potentially emotional issues at the start of a patient visit. However, doctors in our Mindful Medicine group have said that asking these questions at the start of a patient encounter saves you the dreaded experience of having a patient stop you as you are exiting the room and telling you what is really bothering them: a symptom or situation you cannot dismiss that may keep you in the room for another fifteen minutes.

Research indicates that patients' fears center on two themes: loss of control and depersonalization.[43] Illness can make us all feel a loss of control. Just putting on a patient gown can make any of us feel depersonalized and anxious. We have the ability to help with both of these fears by directly asking about a patient's worries, warmly and attentively listening, and reassuring them, when we are able to do so.

FINAL WORDS

Fear is the destroyer of our happiness. Directly asking about it is an important step in healing.

Asking about Sources of Support

THE PRACTICE

Ask patients—or the parents of child patients—what sources of support they have in their lives. If they are confused by the question, you could ask about specifics. Is there anyone you can call on if you need help? Or if you just need to talk to someone? Do you live alone? If so, is there anyone who checks in on you?

REMINDING YOURSELF

Post a note "Sources of support?" where you will see it as a patient encounter begins.

DISCOVERIES

In our outpatient clinics, we don't routinely ask about sources of support. Questions about support are particularly relevant to single parents, teen parents, first-time parents, people with physical disabilities, those who are homeless, the newly divorced, people with chronic physical or mental illness, and elderly people. As I drew up this list, I realized that, unless you are a pricey concierge doctor, it could include most of your patients!

The literature on the beneficial effects of family support for patients describes four potential sources of support: emotional, physical, material, and informational. For example, the adult children of an elderly patient might know how to lift a parent's negative mood, could help prepare meals or make sure medications are being taken, might be able to buy medications that their parents cannot afford, and could take notes during a parent's doctor visit and later read what the doctor said back to their confused parent.

It's easy to add a few questions relevant to these four sources of support and also to add a question about religious or spiritual support. This would help us to be more realistic as we give advice, make treatment recommendations, and prescribe. It could also catalyze compassion when we learn more about our patient's life situation. The references at the end of the book share a sample questionnaire you might give to patients in the waiting room.

An ob-gyn doctor in our group said that she always asks parents with a new baby about sources of support before discharging them from the hospital. After I had knee and cataract surgery, I was asked who would drive me home, but I've never had a doctor or nurse ask about broader sources of support. Has a physician or nurse ever asked you when you were a patient?

Patient and Family-Centered Care (PFCC) is becoming a fundamental concept in medical care in the United States. This movement is led by research clearly documenting the benefits of family and social support for patients with chronic illnesses, such as mental illness, end-stage renal disease, or addiction.

Diabetes presents a clear example. Among the general patient population, 25 percent are found to be nonadherent to treatment. Among people with diabetes, this rises to 50 percent even though there can be severe consequences to vision, kidney, and heart functioning. A meta-analysis of 122 papers showed that adherence was 27 percent higher when patients with diabetes had positive social and family support. In cohesive families—described as warm, accepting, and close—adherence was threefold higher than in families perceived to be non-cohesive. Among patient populations of children and adolescents, 50–70 percent fail to follow treatment recommendations. Thus, conflict between parents and their children who have type 1 diabetes is not rare.[44]

PFCC includes programs that encourage unrestricted visiting hours and enroll family members to participate in some aspects of a patient's care before discharge. For example, nurses may teach patients' family members skills such as dressing changes that they will need to do at home. The benefits are many: decreased pain and anxiety in patients, improved communication between medical staff and patients, faster healing, and decreased length of stay in hospital. Families who could visit anytime or who were involved in caring for their patient/loved ones have reported greater trust in the care being given to their relative and increased ability to cope with their relative's illness even when they are faced with a terminal diagnosis.[45]

The positive effects on patients, families, and nurses applied even when a patient was undergoing a painful procedure in the burn unit, and surprisingly, when the family chose to be present during CPR. In one program, family members were asked if they wanted to stay in the room during a resuscitation, and if so, a staff member was assigned to stand with them and explain what was happening. These self-selected relatives had positive reactions, saying they were grateful to see for themselves that "everything had been done" to try to save the life of their loved one and felt a sense of closure if their loved one died.[46]

Some hospitals have Family Caregiver Programs to involve the family in discharge planning and help link them to a secondary caregiving system, an often ignored but significant source of support to patients and families. This secondary system includes longtime friends, extended family members, neighbors, church groups, and disease-specific support groups. Studies show that these programs can reduce readmissions over the next six months by one-quarter.[47]

It's odd that we send a patient home after a medical encounter or hospital stay, assuming that they will follow our instructions, obtain medications and then take the correct dose at the correct times, and make and keep appointments for physical therapy, consultations with specialists, or additional tests. We do this often not knowing anything about their living conditions or sources of help and support.

When I worked at a small neighborhood clinic in Los Angeles, I discovered that an extended immigrant family of fifteen people lived in a two-bedroom apartment. To me, it seemed like a miracle that everyone could be fed, find a place to sleep, be sent off to school or work on time wearing clean clothes, let alone all use their one bathroom! I gained a tremendous appreciation for their ability to show up with one of their children—clean and nicely dressed—for a scheduled follow-up appointment. When you find out more about some of your patients' lives, your admiration for their strength and perseverance in the face of adversity can't help but grow.

DEEPER LESSONS

In healthcare, we are often timid about asking or talking about religion. Yet, for some people, their religion is a major source of comfort, companionship, and even practical help, as when members bring meals to someone who is ill, newly bereaved, or who just had a baby or surgery. I found only one study that documented religious support, finding that "when the family provides spiritual support and has a strong religious faith, the patient recovery process becomes faster and stronger."[48]

I have a neighbor, a grandmother, who had lived since she married at age eighteen in an area of the city that is now undergoing gentrification. Her husband was fifteen years older than she and died when their daughter was young. When we talk about difficult issues such as police mistreatment of people of color, drug addiction, or the COVID-19 pandemic, she always concludes with, "I just can't worry about these things. I trust in God. He knows what he's doing even if I don't understand it." She goes to church every week and volunteers to help with church outreach missions. Her trust in God's plan is evident in her cheerful, generous outlook on life, despite all the hardships she's faced and witnessed.

Can we find ways to ask about the vital resource of religious or spiritual support and not leave it to the hospital chaplain during a crisis? We could use a questionnaire, or simply ask, "We know that many people get support from their religious or spiritual groups, from prayer, or from meditation. Is that true for you?" If the answer is yes, you could ask, "Can you tell me how that supports you?"

It is important for you, also, to have sources of support. Stop for a moment and list the individuals or groups that help you through difficult times. Consider joining a Mindful Medicine group, in person or online (see chapter 8 for suggestions on starting a group). In an effort to address the stress many healthcare workers feel and to promote more compassionate care, many hospitals offer Schwartz Rounds, a type of grand rounds that provides these professionals a time "to openly and honestly discuss the social and emotional issues they face in caring for patients and families. In contrast to traditional medical rounds, the focus is on the human dimension of medicine. Thus caregivers have an opportunity to share their experiences, thoughts, and feelings on thought-provoking topics drawn from actual patient cases."[49]

There are sources of support beyond that offered by other people. When you meditate or sit in contemplative prayer, you might ponder the question, "What is supporting me at this moment?" We may not know it, but we all live lives of great faith. When we get out of bed in the morning and put our feet down, we have complete faith that the floor will be there to support us. At the same time, we have faith in gravity, that it will continue to pull us toward the earth and we will not float away. We breathe in with complete faith that the air will contain 21 percent oxygen and 78 percent nitrogen. We have faith that our lungs will absorb that oxygen and exhale excess carbon dioxide.

When you begin to investigate what provides support to you at this moment, start with the organs and cells in your own body and expand outward to include objects such as your chair, computer, and house as well as other people who support you. Bring to mind the obvious sources of support (a partner or parent) and the less obvious (the people behind the scenes at the post office, the road repair crew, the garbage truck driver, and the green plants that supply 21 percent oxygen to each breath while depending upon the CO_2 that we breathe out). The answers begin to flow in, expanding to include hundreds of things and people. To be aware of the support that countless beings and objects continually provide you is to begin to realize the truth of interbeing. If all other living beings disappeared, we could not continue to live.

FINAL WORDS

We live in a vast network of unending support. And we are an integral part of that network, continually providing support to people and other beings, including many who will be forever unknown to us.

Asking about Enjoyment or Blessings

THE PRACTICE

Ask patients to list three things that they enjoy in their life. If they give a one-word answer, ask a few follow-up questions. For example, if they say, "exercise," ask what kind of exercise. It could turn out to be anything from running ultra-marathons to gardening to having sex. If they say, "nature," it could involve wilderness survival courses or a TV show about raccoons.[50]

Alternatively, you can ask patients to tell you about three blessings in their lives.

It seems on the surface that it is repetitive to ask patients about what they are grateful for, what they enjoy in life, and what are the blessings in their life. Aren't we asking the same question with different words?

However, when we did these three exercises in our Mindful Medicine group, we found that we had different responses to each of the three "bringing to mind" questions, about gratitude, enjoyment, and blessings. Asking ourselves about what we are grateful for often brought up the simple things that had happened during the day such as a thank-you from a patient or things we often take for granted such as having plenty of food, a bed, and/or a mind that still works. Asking ourselves about three enjoyments in our life brought up activities such as exercise, cooking food for others, or digging in the garden. Asking ourselves about three blessings in our life was likely to bring up relationships (friends, partners, and grandchildren) or something positive that was unexpected.

REMINDING YOURSELF

Tape a note saying "Three things they enjoy or three blessings in their life?" to your computer screen.

DISCOVERIES

This is another way to connect to your patients as unique and interesting people, not just a diagnosis. Asking questions, with genuine curiosity, is a way to help open up a palpable connection with the people who trust that we will do what we can to help them remain healthy and improve their health. The simple questions we ask about enjoyments, hobbies, fears, worries, and pets address our common humanity: human beings who encounter both blessings and difficulties navigating our lives. Both you and they will enjoy a few minutes of talk about enjoyments and blessings before moving on to their current medical difficulties.

You may make discoveries that affect your decisions about healthcare. A pediatric neurologist in our Mindful Medicine group had been seeing teenagers who seemed to be part of an epidemic of unusual motor tics during the COVID-19 pandemic. By asking about activities they enjoyed, she found that the teens spent significant time looking at TikTok, and that they had all seen other teens with motor or verbal tics on that social media app.[51]

You might discover that a patient has a child with autism or a parent with dementia and that, although there are struggles, they count this person as a blessing.[52] One supporting website for parents lists forty blessings of having a child or teen with autism.[53]

A psychiatrist in our group who works with military veterans named telemedicine as a blessing. She said that changing to online sessions had lessened the toll that the stream of human suffering contained in patient encounters had been taking on her own mental health. She enjoyed being able to use little breaks to refresh herself by taking a walk in her garden or fixing a snack in her kitchen. Telemedicine had extended her ability to keep working in her chosen field when she had been close to quitting.

DEEPER LESSONS

If we could see into the future, we might discover that what seems like a difficulty now will transform into a blessing. I worked with a nurse practitioner who was devastated when his partner suddenly announced she wanted to end their relationship. He was noticeably depressed for a year until he met a woman who was a much better match for his personality. It was a delight to witness suffering transformed into a blessing and to see their marriage thrive over the years.

A psychiatrist lost her license after she became involved with a client. This resulted in a period of meditation and introspection in which she realized that her primary task in psychiatry had been to wean patients off unneeded medications to give them back their lives and ability to think clearly. These were patients who were taking a cocktail of many medications due to successive additions by successive doctors. When she completed the requirements of the medical board to regain her license, she looked forward to a new job in the field of addictions and also backward to the hidden blessing contained in an apparent disaster, one that had enabled her to stop and ponder what she really wanted to do.

FINAL WORDS

Make sure that the things you enjoy in life have space on your calendar.

And when something seems to turn out badly, remember that in a few years you may see it as a blessing.

This Person Could Die Tonight

THE PRACTICE

As you greet each patient or client, and as you say goodbye, briefly look them in the eyes and remember that this person could die tonight. This is especially relevant when you know the patient has multiple medical issues.

REMINDING YOURSELF

Put a note on your bathroom mirror saying, "This person could die tonight." Put a less obvious note such as "Gone tonight?" on your workspace computer screen.

DISCOVERIES

This exercise might seem morbid at first, but it helps us remember what we medical people know to be true. Anyone, including us, could die tonight. We have seen proof over and over that the human body is simultaneously very resilient and very fragile. One of our receptionists went home at lunch to check on her middle-aged husband, who had stayed home from work with the flu, and found him in bed and dead. A friend found her apparently healthy ten-year-old son dead in bed when she went to call him to get up for school, probably of viral myocarditis. My cardiologist died of a heart attack while jogging on the beach in Hawaii on vacation.

A certain amount of denial is necessary for us so we don't walk through our days obsessed with death. Once, my husband and I arrived at New Delhi airport at night. We sped through the night toward the city on a road with only occasional dim streetlamps in a taxi with no headlights. We frequently swerved around the carts and sacred cows and trucks on the wrong side of the road that unexpectedly loomed up out of the darkness. The next morning at breakfast, I read in the newspaper that 50 percent of the syringes sold as new in the city pharmacies had been found to have blood residue, indicating they had been pulled out of the hospitals' trash and recycled, in a city with a high incidence of HIV infection. Another story related that a plane at the airport had been rendered inoperable because rats had chewed on the wires in the engine.

As we emerged from the hotel to take a walk, I noticed that a pile of bricks being used to construct a new hotel across the street—the same kind of bricks in the walls of our hotel—was disintegrating in the rain. Returning that night, I blew my nose; the mucus was black from the pollution in the air. I had read travel advisories about not drinking water that had not been boiled in front of your eyes, not using tap water to wash contact lenses for fear of a horrible infection that could destroy the cornea, and not to open your mouth in the shower. The next morning as we left the hotel I thought, "A thousand ways to die today." And, as I returned to the United States, I realized that I've become inured to the risks at home, from social isolation to ubiquitous gun ownership—and actually there are a thousand ways to die today everywhere.

This is always true, but a veil of denial mercifully keeps us from seeing it most of the time and thus being consumed with anxiety. A virus, an inattentive driver in the opposite lane, a slip off a rock while taking a selfie, a hit in the chest by a ball during a baseball game, a fall off a balcony from a rotten railing, a funny "challenge" seen and imitated on social media—healthcare workers and first responders know what most people do not: there are thousands of ways to die unexpectedly. To be aware of this fact and not be overwhelmed with anxiety for ourselves and those we love, we must protect ourselves by ignoring the fact of impermanence.

DEEPER LESSONS

It's important to do this practice not only with our sickest patients but also with everyone, especially those we love, but whose years with us we assume will be many and healthy.

When we are in a hurry, we often only half listen and don't really look at the person we are talking to. When we recognize the truth that either of us could die tonight, our heart opens. We can listen, look, and speak with a clearer awareness of this one unique encounter. When Japanese people say goodbye to a friend, they stand and wave until the car or train is out of sight. They hold the poignant awareness that this could be the last time they will see this person.

People comment that when they bring this awareness to their interactions, irritation and impatience disappear. They are more careful to be fully present as they say goodbye to their partner, children, and friends. How sad would we feel if this were our last moment together and we parted in irritation, anger, or just distraction? This practice is also relevant to bedtimes. The chance that we would awaken and find that someone in our bed or house has died during the night is very low, but if it did happen, it would be nice to have the memory of a last, loving goodnight hug, kiss, or affectionate words.

People also find that when they hold the awareness that this person could die tonight, it brings patience and kindness to encounters with people they previously found annoying. Isn't that interesting, that when we see other people as impermanent and subject—as we all are—to death, their "otherness" evaporates?

We frequently chant the Five Remembrances at the monastery where I live to remind us of the truth of impermanence and the precious nature of this moment and all the moments of our lives.

I am of the nature to grow old. There is no way to escape growing old.

I am of the nature to become ill. There is no way to escape being ill.

I am of the nature to die. There is no way to escape death.

All that is dear to me and everyone I love are of the nature to change. There is no way to escape being separated from them.

My actions are my only true belongings. I cannot escape the consequences of my actions.

My actions are the ground upon which I stand.

When we accept that life could last an hour, a day, or a year, then each moment of life becomes more precious. And when we accept that through the chain of cause and effect, other people will inherit the consequences of our actions, we become more dedicated to living ethically.

FINAL WORDS

Life is not personal, perfect, or permanent.[54]

6

GUIDED MEDITATIONS

Here are a few guided meditations for you to use for your own well-being. (Recordings of these meditations can be found at www.shambhala.com/mindfulmedresources.) Gratitude for the Body, Loving Kindness for the Body, and Discovering and Releasing Tension in the Body can be like a warm bath for your hardworking body. If anyone in your family or one of your patients or clients is interested, you might teach these meditations to them or give them the link to the recordings.

Gratitude for the Body

You can do this guided meditation either sitting or lying down. If you lie down and fall asleep partway through, that's just fine. You need the sleep.

As we do this exercise, we are going to use the mind's awareness like a flashlight, moving it to one body part at a time. This is sometimes called a body scan.

This exercise is a scan of different body parts, with one difference. After you have focused your awareness on a body part, and just before moving on to the next body part, you say silently, "Thank you (name of body part) for _____" and then you leave a blank. Let whatever arises in the mind fill in the blank. If nothing arises, that's OK.

It often helps to close your eyes as it makes focusing your awareness on one body part at a time easier to do. If you are uncomfortable closing your eyes, it is fine to keep them open.

Feet

We begin with the feet. If your eyes are closed and you cannot see your feet, how do you know that there are feet at the ends of your legs? What are the sensations arising from the feet? Perhaps you are aware of pressure, or tingling, or sensations of warmth or coolness. Hold your awareness on these sensations for a while as they arise, persist, and then fade away. (pause)

Then say silently, "Thank you, feet, for _____."

Pause and see if anything arises in that blank space. If nothing arises in the gap, that's OK.

Stomach

Now move your awareness to your stomach, wherever you feel your stomach to be. How do you know you have a stomach? What are the physical sensations arising from your stomach? Perhaps there are sensations of pressure, fullness, warmth, or coolness, or there might even be sounds. Be aware of these sensations as they arise, persist, and then fade away. Rest your awareness in your stomach for a while. (pause)

Then, before moving on to another body part, you silently say, "Thank you, stomach, for _____." Pause and see if anything arises. If not, that's OK.

Heart

Now move your awareness to your heart, your physical heart. How do you know you have a heart? What are the physical sensations arising from your heart? Perhaps you feel movement or pressure or hear sounds. Be aware of these sensations as they arise, persist, and then fade away. Rest your awareness in your heart for a while. (pause)

Then, before moving on to another body part, you silently say, "Thank you, heart, for _____." Pause to see if anything arises. If not, that's OK. (pause)

Please continue to move your mind's awareness to different body parts. After you've rested in your awareness of the sensations from that body part, arising and disappearing, remember to say, "Thank you for . . ." and see if words or thoughts arise in that gap.

Before ending the meditation, move your awareness to a body part that is having some difficulty or isn't functioning as well as you would like it to. Are there any sensations arising from that body part? Perhaps there is a sense of warmth or coolness, tingling, light or firm pressure, moisture or dryness, pain, or even movement. Be aware of these sensations as they arise, persist, and then fade away. Rest your awareness in that body part for a while.

Now silently say, "Thank you (name of body part) for ____," and see if anything arises. If not, that's OK. (pause)

Ending

Now, as we finish, if your eyes are closed, let them gently open.

Note: With non-medical people, we do this exercise with the feet, stomach, heart, mouth, eyes, brain, and body fat. Medical people have knowledge and awareness of many more body parts than non-medical folks. That means you have lots of parts you could include such as the liver, pancreas, spleen, kidneys, reproductive organs, thyroid, or glottis. Your medical specialty may affect what you include—neurosurgeons might add the hypothalamus and orthopedists might include the joint capsules and joint fluid.

QUESTIONS

1. Did anything arise to fill in the blank when you silently said, "Thank you for ____"?
2. Were you surprised by some words or thoughts that appeared in that blank space?

Loving Kindness for the Body

You can do this guided meditation either sitting or lying down. If you lie down and fall asleep partway through, that's just fine. You need the sleep.

It is especially important to do this meditation if your body parts are not functioning as well as you would like. When we are sick, or an organ is having difficulties, it is easy to slide into a negative attitude toward that part of our body, annoyance, or even anger. Nothing can thrive in an environment of negative thoughts and emotions—not our partners, our children, our patients, our pets, nor even our plants. This meditation is an antidote for this phenomenon.

As we do this exercise, we are going to use the mind's awareness like a flashlight, moving it to one body part at a time. This is sometimes called a body scan.

This exercise is similar to Gratitude for the Body, with one difference. As you bring awareness to each body part, we send it loving kindness (metta or maitri). Traditional metta practice involves saying the following phrases, directing them first toward oneself, then moving outward in ever-widening circles to include the entire universe.

May you be free from suffering.
May you be at ease.
May you be happy.

In this case, we direct the phrases inward, toward the parts of our body, the inhabitants of our inner universe. Here are examples of phrases to direct to body parts, on the out-breath. Please create your own phrases according to the condition of your body.

May you (a body part or organ) be(come) free from tension, distress, disease, or pain.

May you (aware of a body part or organ) be(come) healthy and function as well as you are able.

May you (aware of a body part or organ) be at ease.

You can begin at the top of your body, with your scalp or your brain, and move down, or at the bottom, with your toes and move up. You can bring different body parts into awareness on different days.

Discovering and Releasing
Tension in the Body

———

You can do this exercise either sitting—even at your desk—or lying down, as a way to prepare for sleep.

Begin by taking three deep breaths. Breathe in, briefly hold it, and then let it go, extending the length of the out-breath somewhat, in a way that is comfortable for you. Starting at the top of your body, do a body scan at your own speed, bringing awareness to parts of the body that seem to accumulate and/or store tension or tightness.

Begin by bringing awareness to the scalp. Be curious. Is there any extra holding or tension in your scalp? If so, can you soften or release it a bit on the out-breath? Now move your awareness to your forehead. Investigate. Is there any extra holding or tension in your forehead? If so, gently release it on the out-breath. Now move your awareness to the space between your eyebrows. Wiggle your eyebrows a little. Then soften that area on the out-breath.

Next, move your awareness to the area around your eyes. Let it soften or relax on the out-breath. (There is research showing that when you soften this area, your brain waves change to a meditative pattern.) Now become aware of your lips. Are they pressed together? Let them soften, perhaps turning the edges up a bit into a faint smile.

Continue this pattern. Here are areas of the body not to miss: your jaw, the back of your neck, your shoulders, your hands, your belly, your lower back, and your feet.

Sometimes when I do this as I lie down at night, I quickly scan through a second time and discover that a few areas have become tight again—this unconscious tension is so habitual! I might need to do the scan three times before my body feels truly relaxed, yielding into the support of the bed.

Grounding Your Mind in the Earth

———

This meditation is based upon how we ground electricity in the earth to keep ourselves safe from an excess of energy that could harm us. When our minds are too full of churning thoughts and difficult emotions, we can ground that energy, the excess electricity running through the overactive neural networks of our brain, into the earth and thus refresh our minds.

You can do this exercise sitting or standing up. I like to do it standing up, first because my feet have more solid contact with the floor and also because there are many times during the day when I am standing. I can ground my mind in the earth when I'm waiting in line at the hospital cafeteria or the grocery store, when I'm standing in an elevator, or when I'm standing waiting for surgery to commence.

If you do it sitting down, you might take off your shoes for a few minutes to increase the contact with the ground. You can do it seated in a meeting if your mind becomes restless. You know those meetings where they could have tape-recorded the last meeting and just played it back and saved everyone a lot of time? One of those meetings. It's also one of many ways to clear your mind between patients. When you are standing at the exam room door or looking at the chart, ground and clear your mind.

Begin by becoming aware of your feet, the ankles, the tops of the feet, the arch, the toes, and then the bottoms of the feet. Notice the places where the bottoms of your feet are in stronger contact with the floor (through your shoes). Moving your attention down through the floor, become aware of the earth that is underneath the floor and the foundation of the building you are in. The earth is always supporting you, unfailing in its support, whether you notice it or not. The earth pulls you toward it, securely holding you down so you don't float away. When we get out of bed in the morning, we put our feet on the floor without hesitation, completely trusting that continuous holding, that continuous support.

Now bringing your awareness to your mind, wherever you feel your mind to be. Gather up all the thoughts and emotions in your mind into a ball. Let that ball smoothly move down through your body, out the bottoms of your feet, and into the earth. The earth will absorb and disperse this like it does water.

Check your mind again. Is it still full of the energy of swirling thoughts? You can package it all up again and let it move down through your body into the earth. You may need to do this a few more times before you feel that your mind has noticeably settled down.

The more often you practice this mind-clearing exercise, the easier it becomes to notice and settle your restless mind.

Dissolving Skin

Imagine yourself and everyone else with transparent skin. This appearance will be familiar to you from anatomy illustrations in which the first layer, skin, has been removed, revealing a body of flesh, tendons, bones, nerves, and blood vessels.

BACKGROUND FOR THIS PRACTICE

This is a meditation on skin, but it has the potential of becoming much more.

This exercise came from four sources. First, I am interested in how vision affects our assessment and treatment of others. If you carefully watch your mind, you will notice that when you meet a stranger, your mind makes an instant assessment based upon their skin color and condition, general cleanliness, whether they have missing, discolored or decaying teeth, and many other aspects including clothing, the length and styling or messiness of their hair, whether they wear glasses, their body shape and weight, and their overall attractiveness according to current beauty standards.

When I was about twelve years old, I became curious about how blind people negotiated their way in the world. Did they have internal maps of familiar terrain? What navigation cues did they use? Did the sense of hearing become more acute when not distracted by a complex visual field? Could a kind of radar evolve based upon subtle echoes from walls and furniture? I was very curious about how my first impressions of people were based on visual cues. I wondered how blind people formed their initial judgments of a person; perhaps on the sound of their voice or their smell?

Some Saturdays, I wore a blindfold for several hours to investigate these questions. I discovered that it was helpful to count how many steps there were in the stairs up to my second-story bedroom or from our front porch down to the ground. Counting enabled me to climb or descend with more confidence, instead of waving a tentative foot in the air, feeling for the next stair. I found that eating was a messy business when I was "blind." I became much more sensitive to sound.

The second source for this meditation on dissolving skin came from practicing ancient Buddhist meditations on the thirty-two parts of the body, which begin with contemplating your skin, nails, and teeth. You open your awareness to one body part at a time.

The third source is educational exhibits such as Body Worlds, where plasticized human bodies are displayed without skin, showing us the universal and complex beauty that is everyone's body.[1]

The fourth source was hearing stories of daily aggression against my friends and students who are people of color. I pondered how not being able to see skin color and hair might affect the damage of ongoing prejudice in our country, prejudice that, of course, also exists in my mind.

THE MEDITATION

Sit in a comfortable position. Lower or close your eyes.

Bringing your attention now to your entire body, this body that sits and breathes. Let your attention rest in your body for at least a few breaths.

Now release your attention from the entire body and bring it to focus your skin, the skin that envelops your body. If you cannot see your skin, how do you know that you have skin? Spend a minute or two becoming aware of the sensations coming from your skin. Perhaps there are sensations of temperature, more coolness or warmth in certain areas? Perhaps there are sensations of touch, like the movement of clothing against your body as you breathe? Perhaps there is a tingling, like millions of tiny touches all over the body?

Sit for a few minutes with your full awareness on the skin bag that encloses and protects your body. Now imagine that your skin seems to dissolve or disappear, leaving your body safely enclosed in a thin, flexible, completely transparent covering. You are visible simply as a body of flesh, muscle, tendons, and bones, nerves and blood vessels, like the pictures in anatomy books.

Next, imagine that your hair and nails (which are outgrowths of your skin) also disappear. All the hair on your head and body and also your finger and toenails disappear. When you look in a mirror, this is what you see: a body without skin, hair, or nails. What would change about your self-image if you are a body without hair and skin? If you are just a body of flesh, muscles, tendons, and bones?

What happens to the judgments of your Inner Critic about your body when you look in the mirror and you see no hair nor skin, just a body of flesh and muscles connected by sinews to bones?

Expand this new awareness to other people, your family, coworkers, and patient, so they also have no skin. They are all just bodies of flesh, muscles, tendons, and bones. Sitting, walking around, interacting, as bodies without skin.

Does this make a difference in how you see and relate to other people? A difference in sexual attraction?

Imagine greeting a patient or client in the exam room or in your office. Both of you have no hair or skin. Would this make a difference in your interaction?

Now imagine everyone in the world without skin or hair. Would this make a difference in the problems of prejudice and discrimination in the world?[2]

Bring your attention back to your body, to the sensations of a body, clothed in skin, that is sitting or lying down. Open your awareness to include the room around you, the walls, ceiling, and furniture in the room. Now, when you are ready, if your eyes are closed, let them gently open.

7

RESCUE REMEDIES FOR
TIMES OF ACUTE NEED

When we are under the most stress, when we are working hard without a break, that is the very time we need to "increase the dose" of the medicine that will help us remain—or restore ourselves to being—centered, clear-minded, and compassionate. It is also a time when most healthcare workers cannot afford to take thirty minutes to meditate in the silence of a meditation hall or even at home.

Here are some very brief practices that busy healthcare and mental health workers and emergency responders can use while at work when they detect that anxiety is arising and interfering with their ability to focus and work quickly and efficiently. These are practices that can quickly help the mind stop spinning, provide mental refreshment, and bring us back to a place of internal balance.

I suggest that you try each one a few times and find the ones that work best for you.

4-7-8 Relaxation Breathing

We've all had the experience of releasing tension by forcefully sighing or exhaling. This is a refinement of that natural action.

Place your tongue on the roof of your mouth with the tip pressing against the gum ridge behind the upper front teeth.

> Fully breathe out.
> Breathe in through your nose as you silently count from one to four.
> Hold your breath as you count from one to seven.
> Breath out through your mouth as you count from one to eight. You can purse your lips to control the outward flow and make a "whooshing" sound.
> Repeat for four full breaths.

You can count at your own rate. Do this for four breaths and then resume normal, unregulated breathing. Notice any effects on the body, heart, or mind.

This is one of the most potent Rescue Remedies for helping the mind return to its natural clear, calm state. It is based upon pranayama yogic breathing, which activates the parasympathetic nervous system, relaxing the body and calming the mind. Dr. Andrew Weil recommends doing four breaths twice a day and gradually advancing to eight breaths twice a day.[1] Studies show that 4-7-8 breathing can reduce depression and anxiety and reduce blood pressure and migraine symptoms.[2]

Brief Body Scan

Begin by finding a comfortable seated posture. You can also do this standing up if you are still, as when waiting.

This is a short version of the usual body scan. You will be moving the light of your awareness down through your body like the descent of a warm healing liquid, from your scalp to your toes. Pick your own speed depending on your circumstances and time restraints. You can do it in several long breaths or take a luxurious three minutes.

Start by bringing your awareness to your scalp. On the out-breath, slowly move your attention down your body. Pause on the in-breath. As the warm healing liquid of awareness descends through your body, it softens any extra holding or tension and brings a sense of well-being.

Be especially aware of tension in the forehead between and around the eyes, around the mouth or in the jaw, in the neck and shoulders, or within the belly and the back.

When you finish your three breaths or three minutes of body scanning, envelop your entire body in a cocoon of warm awareness for another three breaths. Before you end, thank your body for how it has served you this day.

Regular use of the body scan meditation has been shown to decrease stress and symptoms of mental illness, reduce biological markers and subjective ratings of stress, increase perception of personal well-being, improve the quality of sleep, and reduce distress related to chronic pain.[3]

Breathing Peace

———

This is a very simple practice, one that is easy to summon up in any situation.

As you breathe in, you silently say, "Peace." As you breathe out, you silently say, "Peace." You can change the words to suit the situation. You could use words like *ease*, *love*, or *serenity*. Try turning up the corners of your mouth in a very slight smile as you do this practice.

The Zen master Thich Nhat Hanh taught this version: "Breathing in, I calm body and mind. Breathing out, I smile. Dwelling in the present moment, I know this is the only moment."

Listen to the Sound of Silence

You know how it is when you are on a long drive and you realize that you've heard the same news stories three times already and you reach over and turn off the radio? And the sound of silence is so lovely?

When you discover that your mind is compulsively playing the same unpleasant thoughts over and over, imagine that you reach up into your brain and intentionally turn off the obsessive thinking station. Tune in to a peaceful station instead, the one that was covered up by the noise in your head. It's the lovely sound of silence.

At first, you have to hold on to it a bit. But after a while, the resting mind—the mind of awareness, instead of the mind filled with thoughts—becomes your fallback, your refuge. It also becomes the source of sudden flashes of insight and wisdom.

Mantra

Mantra means "mind release." Mantras are intended to release the turmoil of thoughts, quieting and focusing one's mind, bringing it to a state of restful awareness. Mantras substitute beneficial words or phrases for the tangle of thoughts in a stressed and anxious mind. If you hold your attention on the mantra, it prevents the mind from ruminating over difficulties in the past or spinning about possible disasters in the future.

Mantras can be chanted silently or out loud, depending upon your circumstances. You can vary the speed of the chanting until you find the pace that works best to quiet and calm the mind. If your mind is anxious, you can try speeding up the recitation, then slowing it down as your mind settles. When the mind is calmer, you can try saying the mantra on the out-breath and resting in quiet mind during the in-breath.

People who regularly do mantra practice regard it as a spiritual practice, saying that it calls forth certain beneficial energies within your own being and in the world. You can use any word or phrase from any language or tradition. "Grant me wisdom and compassion for those in pain." "May all lives be uplifted and blessed." "*Dona nobis pacem,*" "*Nada te turbe, nada te espante,*" "*Ubi caritas et amor, Deus ibi est.*"[4]

Here are two mantras you might try:

The first is a mantra invoking Kuan Yin, the archetype in Asia of one who hears the cries of all those who suffer in this world and responds with compassion.

OM MANE PADME HUM

The second is a mantra invoking Jizo Bodhisattva, the archetype in Asia of the benevolent guardian of those who are vulnerable or need extra help as they negotiate their particular life path, including women and children.[5] The other qualities attributed to Jizo are great benevolence, great determination, great optimism, fearlessness, and a clear life vow or life purpose.

OM KA KA KABI SAN MA EI SOWA KA

Meditation practices involving mantra have been shown to decrease high blood pressure and psychological distress (using scales of anxiety, anger, depression, fatigue, and confusion) and increase self-reported quality of life.[6] They have been successful in reducing symptoms of post-traumatic stress disorder in African refugees and American veterans of conflict in the Middle East.[7]

Empty like the Room

Ordinarily, we only pay attention to the physical objects in a room—the rugs, furniture, and people. In this exercise, you purposely open your awareness to the space in the room.

There is more space in a room than stuff, almost always. Notice the stuff and then do a figure-ground reversal. Reverse your attention from the contents of the room you are in to all the empty space in that room. Hold your awareness in that space and invite that same space into your mind so your mind also becomes empty and spacious. Enjoy the sense of freedom from the inner chatter of thoughts. Soon, they will fill up your mind again, but once you have consistently practiced this exercise, when thoughts become annoying or stressful, you will always be able to let them go and refresh your mind in this way.

Grounding Your Mind in the Earth:
Short Version

———

This is a short version of the guided meditation Grounding Your Mind in the Earth. You can do this grounding—a pause that refreshes—while standing or as you sit in your office.

If you become aware that your mind is agitated and unclear or you are becoming angry, immediately direct your mind's attention to your feet. Feel the support of the floor and extend that sense of support all the way down into the earth.

The Buddha pointed out that the earth receives anything we throw on it without complaint: blood, pus, clean water, vomit, honey, urine, and feces.[8] In medicine, many things can be thrown into our heart-minds, both literally and figuratively.

The earth has witnessed countless wars and epidemics and received millions of bodies into its embrace. And still, days and nights trade places, spring comes, trees put forth new leaves, flowers bloom, and bees gather nectar. Can you feel the equanimity of the earth, how it continually supports you, wherever you go? Can you breathe in that stability, that equanimity, up from the ground, into your own being?

Brief Gratitude Practice

This is a brief version of Actively Practicing Gratitude in chapter 4.

In the midst of a charged and chaotic workplace, when you notice that you are feeling frazzled, briefly pause and open your mind's awareness, searching for at least three things you are grateful for in this place at this moment. You might find more than three. (You can do this so no one notices, for example, while taking a few extra minutes as you look at the electronic chart, while washing your hands, in a short pause before eating, or even in the bathroom—which might be the only place all day that you have a few free minutes.)

I'll give you an example: I close my eyes—and I become aware of my heart beating in my chest. I am grateful that it has been faithfully beating all day and night since before I was born. I notice sensations of my clothing touching my skin. I am grateful for the people who made the clothing that keeps me warm in winter. I hear someone vacuuming in the hall. I am grateful for the people who keep the place I live and work clean.

Mindful Self-Compassion: Short Version

———

This is a short version of the Mindful Self-Compassion practice in chapter 4. As soon as you realize that you are distressed, do this:

Say to yourself, "I'm having a hard time." "I'm feeling (anxious, sad, upset, disappointed, etc.)."

Gently touch yourself as a good friend would do, maybe a pat on the arm, a touch on your hand.

Say to yourself, "I'm always here for you."

Take a few deep breaths, prolonging the exhale a bit.

Repeat as needed.

Silly Walking

Silly walking in my experience is one of the easiest and quickest ways to change from a heavy to a lighter mood. That said, there are appropriate places and times to do a silly walk. Maybe not in the administrative wing of the hospital or in a patient room. Try it out at home first and then in an empty corridor or stretch of sidewalk.

The easiest kinds of silly walking are walking backward, skipping, hopping on one foot, or exaggeratedly lifting the knees. You could go upstairs weaving from side to side. Silly walking works because body and mind are not two. It also lightens the mood of observers. See if your kids will do it with you, particularly when they are in an unhappy mood.

Do be careful. We had a resident who tried the Monty Python–inspired galloping, backward, complete with hollow-coconut sound effects.[9] It was very funny to watch until he fell and bruised his elbow.

8

SUGGESTIONS FOR MINDFUL
MEDICINE GROUPS AND RETREATS

Our Mindful Medicine PDX group was created in 2013 by and for medical professionals. It developed in response to the growing pressures and demands of our local healthcare professions, but has expanded to include participants from adjoining states. The founders were three physicians who had benefited from mindfulness training in combination with two therapists who taught Mindfulness-Based Stress Reduction (MBSR).[1] They conferred and decided to focus on bringing mindfulness practices to physicians, reasoning that "if doctors were doing well, then their patients and colleagues would all benefit."

Aware that their "target population" would want evidence for such an undertaking, they reviewed the existing literature. One physician obtained a grant from his hospital system to fund research on the program. The study was small but randomized and controlled. Participants in the Mindful Medicine Curriculum group reported significant improvements in stress ($p < .001$), mindfulness ($p = .05$), emotional exhaustion ($p = .004$), and depersonalization ($p = .01$) whereas in the control group, there were no improvements on these outcomes. At three months, follow-up participants had been able to maintain a regular mindfulness and/or meditation practice with minimal support.[2]

The course included a non-residential weekend retreat with a schedule that was light enough to include time for the doctors to take care of themselves, connect with their families, and answer urgent calls. There were two additional two-hour meetups at two and four weeks post retreat, which were called "booster shots." Currently, there are two weekend retreats a year, with a one-hour evening drop-in meeting once a week.

The curriculum includes brief practical skills drawn from two evidence-based curricula, Mindfulness-Based Stress Reduction and Mindful Self-Compassion, and aspects of the Mindful Practice curriculum.[3] Concepts of professional isolation, moral injury, and trauma are introduced along with vital prevention and self-care skills. Evaluations from the past seven years have shown that there are lasting benefits of combining peer-to-peer connection with mindfulness strategies for reducing stress.

Our mission has expanded to include other medical professionals. We have witnessed deep respect and appreciation for the different ways people serve in the healthcare professions and the common problems they face. We now have nurse practitioners, nurses, dentists, veterinarians, therapists, and acupuncturists participating from several states and time zones. The organization became a nonprofit a few years ago, which was an important decision because it allows Mindful Medicine PDX to be independent of any healthcare system and be completely dedicated to the well-being of all healthcare professionals.

THE BENEFIT OF TALKING TOGETHER

Healthcare professionals are so busy at work that we seldom have time to talk to each other at all—let alone about deep topics. Our brief conversations are usually about puzzling patients, procedures, test results, the latest directive from the administration, and new therapies on the horizon. We don't have time to talk about our grief over the death of a ten-year-old we've come to love, who's been in and out of the hospital with a series of cancer treatments since they were five, and whose family we've supported through the hopes and disappointments of each new treatment regime.

We don't have time to share our distress about turning off life support on the eighteen-year-old killed by a stray bullet in a hot summer drive-by shooting, who in one month would have become the first person in their family to go to college. One curse or prayer under our breath and we move on to the asthmatic patient struggling to breathe in the next bay. Or the twitching, anxious young man with a huge area of cellulitis from skin-popping methamphetamine. Or the woman in ketoacidosis because she can't afford her insulin and was shifted to a new provider whom she cannot see for two months because we don't have universal healthcare in a country founded on life, liberty, and the pursuit of happiness. Mindful Medicine groups provide a place where we can safely express, and thus lighten the burden, of what has lodged in the recesses of our heart as we serve in the trenches of human suffering.

The therapists who colead our Mindful Medicine group meetings have observed that "breakout groups are the secret sauce" of our online meetings. It's true. It's one of the things we discovered during the COVID-19 pandemic, when healthcare professionals began using Zoom to meet regularly and talk openly together about their joys and sorrows, their difficult emotions and difficult patients, and their fantasies about quitting the profession and living in a cabin in the woods, far from a crowded appointment calendar that allows eleven minutes per patient. Just talking together about our challenges, discovering that we are not alone, begins to dissolve distress.

PRACTICAL SUGGESTIONS

Here are some practical suggestions for founding, facilitating, and supporting a Mindful Medicine group.

Meet online for one hour in the evening once a week

Picking a day in the middle of the week avoids Monday overwhelm and Friday exhaustion. The hours of 7–8 p.m. or 8–9 p.m. give people time to take care of things at home before the meeting and still be able to get to bed at a reasonable time.

After a long day of work, fixing dinner, getting kids settled with homework or in bed, and a quick kiss for your partner, traveling to and from an in-person Mindful Medicine meeting wasn't something most healthcare professionals could fit in their week or that relieved stress more than briefly. When we shifted to meeting online for one hour a week, the groups became more cohesive, open, and intimate.

Drop-in basis

Let people know they can drop in as their schedule allows. Don't worry if you have five people one week and ten the next.

Welcome anyone who works on the front lines of healthcare

This includes doctors, nurses, dentists (who also have a high suicide rate), nurse practitioners, nurse midwives, and physician assistants. It could also include emergency medical responders, veterinarians, physicians who are now administrators, and therapists.

Have a topic or mindfulness practice for the week, and an agenda with a time schedule for each component of the hour

Always include group discussion (if your group is five or less) or breakout groups (if your group is larger than five). It creates a palpable feeling of friendship. Here's a sample schedule:

> 5 minutes: Greeting people as they join, introductions all around anytime a new person arrives.
>
> 7 minutes: A guided session of stretches in your chair and a brief meditation to anchor in the body and settle in.
>
> 5 minutes: introduce the topic for the breakout groups.
>
> 20–25 minutes: Breakout groups of 2–3 people. Groups of two give more time for each person to speak; groups of three can reduce pressure to speak.
>
> 10 minutes: Return from the breakout groups and share feedback about any discoveries.
>
> 5 minutes: Introduce a Mindful Medicine practice for the upcoming week.
>
> 3 minutes: Relevant poem? Goodbyes.

Topics for discussion or breakout groups

There are many possibilities. You can use the Mindful Medicine practices in this book, taking up a practice like washing your mind as you wash your hands for a week or two. The discussion could be about discoveries made while doing this practice. After you've tried out ten or twelve weeks of different practices, the group will have found and may request their favorites. The group can also suggest things they'd like to talk about. Some topics we've found especially lively include: How do I care for myself after a hectic week? What my Inner Critic says to me. What sustains me in my work? Why did I go into medicine/first responder work? What instance of moral injury and moral injury residue have I encountered in medicine? The patient I will never forget. What are the quick Rescue Remedies I use to clear my heart and mind between patients?

Facilitation

Our facilitators, both for our weekly online meeting and our in-person weekend retreats, are well-trained experienced MBSR teachers who are also therapists. A person who is currently active or retired from healthcare can be a helpful cofacilitator. The facilitators must be experienced meditators and dedicated mindfulness practitioners, people who walk what they talk.

Duration

This depends upon many factors. You could have a group that meets for just six months, for nine months and takes the summer off, or continues for years. It depends upon whether the group offers what the participants find helpful. Don't confuse participants with irregular schedules. They need to know they can attend when the need arises, often acutely.

Weekend Retreats

These are essential! Over and over, people tell us they were ready to quit medicine or even contemplating suicide and the weekend retreat was a turning point, enabling them to continue in their profession with a tool belt of practices to antidote the stresses that are part of work that immerses you in the various realms of human suffering.

We hold weekend retreats twice a year. Continuing education units are provided by a local hospital. The retreat is purposely non-residential so a participant can attend the entire retreat and still have personal time on Saturday and Sunday mornings for breakfast with the family, chores, exercise, or recreation.

Retreat Schedule Overview
Each day integrates meditation with practicing useful mindfulness skills and contemplative conversations about topics relevant to medical practice.

Friday Evening: 7 p.m.–9 p.m.
- Introductions of teachers and participants
- Introduction to mindfulness practice
- Contemplative conversation topic facilitated by Mindful Medicine leader

Saturday: 10 a.m.–5 p.m.
- Classic formal and informal mindfulness practices
- Contemplative conversation topic facilitated by Mindful Medicine leader
- Working with the challenging patient
- Lunch together beginning with a five-minute Mindful Eating exercise

Sunday: 1 p.m.–5 p.m.
- Heart-opening yoga practice
- Inner Critic, compassion, and self-compassion

- Finding what went well: appreciative inquiry—an antidote to morbidity and mortality conferences
- Contemplative conversation topic facilitated by Mindful Medicine leader
- Intentional self-care goal-setting
- Closing ceremony

Financial Support

Our nonprofit depends upon donations and a fee for the weekend retreat. The current retreat fee is $400 for physicians and dentists, $275 for nurses and other healthcare providers, and $200 for medical residents. No one is turned away for lack of funds. The two therapists who led the retreat are compensated; everyone else is a volunteer including the lunch cook.

Other Models

The University of Rochester Medical School has been training medical students, residents, and physicians in an evidence-based mindful practice curriculum since 2007. They offer workshops and retreats in the United States and internationally.[4]

Stanford University offers events through their WellMD and WellPhD Program including monthly Physician Wellness Forums.[5]

When you search online for "mindful medicine," you will find practitioners, medical and therapy groups, and even cannabis dispensaries that are labeled as "mindful." There are also a few companies that offer consultation and training to help organizations introduce mindfulness into healthcare settings.

Resources, References, and Additional Reading

There are several websites begun by doctors to help other doctors and medical professionals remain healthy in their professions. This one includes many videos and other tools on recognizing and treating burnout, communicating with difficult patients, and effectively communicating with administrators while avoiding being labeled "disruptive."
https://www.thehappymd.com

This site recommends six doctor-to-doctor websites including a site for doctor-moms and a satirical medical news site that will get you laughing.
https://weatherbyhealthcare.com/blog/physician-online-resources

The pages following have sample questionnaires to use with your patients. Downloadable, printable versions of these worksheets are available at www.shambhala.com/mindfulmedresources.

SAMPLE QUESTIONNAIRES TO USE WITH PATIENTS

Questionnaire about Hobbies

Patient's name: _____

Date of birth: _____

Do you have any hobbies? For example, what do you like to do in your free time?

These are my hobbies: _____
_____

Please circle the things you do in your free time from the list below.

Playing an instrument

Listening to music

Reading

Writing

Participating in a team or
 solo sport

Watching movies, TV shows,
 or sports

Listening to podcasts or
 audiobooks

Outdoor activities (hiking,
 bird-watching, etc.)

Gardening

Exercising

Photography

Painting or drawing

Volunteering

Crafting or building

Gaming (video games, board
 games, etc.)

Other

Questionnaire about Sources of Support

Name _____

Date _____

We would like to ask you a few questions about sources of support in your life.

Please fill this questionnaire out and give it to your healthcare provider.

Is there anyone you can call on for help? For example, if you need help with transportation, grocery shopping, or getting medication, or if you had a fall at home or a medical problem.
Check anyone who could help you.

___ My spouse or partner

___ A member of my family

___ A friend

___ A member of my church, temple, or mosque

___ My social worker

___ There is no one I could call to help

Do you live alone? Y/N
If yes, is there anyone who regularly checks up on you, by phone or in person? Y/N
If yes, who is that person? Circle all that apply:
Friend/family member/healthcare, visiting nurse, social worker, or mental healthcare worker.
How do you usually get to your medical visits or tests? Circle the answer(s).

My own car/another person gives me a ride in their car/by bus, taxi, walk, or transport vehicle

Is it easy for you to arrange transportation to your medical visits or tests? Y/N

How do you get your groceries? Circle the answer(s).
Shop myself/someone shops for me/order online.

Can you afford to pay for the medication we prescribe for you? Y/N

Do you belong to any groups that provide support to you? Y/N
If yes, what is that group? Club/group of friends/community group

Do you belong to a group that provides religious or spiritual support to you? Y/N
If yes, please circle the group.
Church/synagogue/temple/mosque/prayer group/Bible study group/meditation group/other.

Notes

INTRODUCTION

1. National Academy of Medicine, *Taking Action Against Clinician Burnout: A Systems Approach to Professional Well-Being* (Washington, DC: The National Academies Press, 2019), 1–3. https://doi.org/10.17226/25521.

   The term *burnout* was invented by a psychologist in the 1970s to describe the results of severe stress and high ideals in the "helping" professions. Burnout is described by the National Academy of Medicine as "a workplace syndrome that is characterized by emotional exhaustion, high depersonalization (i.e., cynicism), and a low sense of personal accomplishment from work.

   Symptoms include irritability and negativity with patients and coworkers and emotional distancing or numbing. Burnout is not a medical diagnosis but is mentioned in the ICD-11 as a problem "resulting from chronic workplace stress that has not been successfully managed." Although many medical workplaces are recognizing burnout, often their remedies, such as after-work seminars on how to "manage" burnout, increase rather than reduce stress by asking healthcare professionals to add another obligation to a day that is already more than full.

2. Pauline Anderson, "Physicians Experience Highest Suicide Rate of Any Profession," Medscape, May 7, 2018, https://www.medscape.com/view article/896257.

3. The Doctors Company, "The Future of Healthcare: A National Survey of Physicians," accessed Nov 25, 2021, https://www.thedoctors.com/about -the-doctors-company/newsroom/the-future-of-healthcare-survey.

4. Ruderman Family Foundation, "Study: Police Officers and Firefighters Are More Likely to Die by Suicide than in Line of Duty," accessed Nov 25, 2021, https://rudermanfoundation.org/white_papers/police-officers-and-fire fighters-are-more-likely-to-die-by-suicide-than-in-line-of-duty/.

5. A state of flow is characterized by complete focus on an activity, unusual clarity, absence of the sense of self, feelings of serenity or even ecstasy, lack of awareness of physical needs, and loss of the sense of time.

A TED Talk by Mihaly Csikszentmihalyi, whose research on flow states opened an entire field of study in positive psychology, can be found here: Mihaly Csikszentmihalyi, "Flow, the Secret of Happiness," *TED*, February 2004, https://www.ted.com/talks/mihaly_csikszentmihalyi_flow_the _secret_to_happiness#t-883527. See also the references in this article: Kendra Cherry, "The Psychology of Flow," *Verywellmind*, https://www.verywell mind.com/what-is-flow-2794768.

CHAPTER 1: BENEFITS OF MINDFULNESS FOR HEALTHCARE PROFESSIONALS

1. About Jon Kabat Zinn, accessed Nov 25, 2021, https://mbsrtraining.com /jon-kabat-zinn/.

2. Renee A. Sheepers et al., "The Impact of Mindfulness-Based Interventions on Doctors' Well-Being and Performance: A Systematic Review," *Medical Education* 54, no. 2 (December 2019): 138–49, https://doi.org/10.1111 /medu.14020.

3. Mary C. Beach et al., "A Multicenter Study of Physician Mindfulness and Health Care Quality," *The Annals of Family Medicine* 11, no. 5 (2013): 421–28, https://doi.org/10.1370/afm.1507.

4. Daniel S. Tawfik et al., "Physician burnout, well-being, and work unit safety grades in relationship to reported medical errors," *Mayo Clinic Proceedings* 93, no. 11 (2018): 1571–80, https://doi.org/10.1016/j.mayocp .2018.05.014.

5. Tawfik et al., "Physician burnout, well-being, and work unit safety grades in relationship to reported medical errors."

6. Tawfik et. al, "Physician burnout, well-being, and work unit safety grades in relationship to reported medical errors."

7. J. Johnson Zeller et al., "Mindfulness Training to Improve Nurse Clinical Performance: A Pilot Study," *Western Journal of Nursing Research* 43, no. 3 (2021): 250–60, https://doi.org/10.1177/0193945920964938.

8. Sheepers et al., "The Impact of Mindfulness-Based Interventions on Doctors' Well-Being and Performance: A Systematic Review," 146.

CHAPTER 2: THE INNER CRITIC IN MEDICINE AND IN LIFE

1. See: Richard G. Gardner et al., "'I Must Have Slipped through the Cracks Somehow': An Examination of Coping with Perceived Impostorism and the Role of Social Support," *Journal of Vocational Behavior* 115 (2019): 103337, https://doi.org/10.1016/j.jvb.2019.103337.

2. For more information on Voice Dialogue and Voice Therapy, see these websites: https://voicedialogueinternational.com and https://www.glendon .org/post-topic/voice-therapy.

3. For more resources on the Inner Critic see: Hal and Sidra Stone, *Embracing Your Inner Critic:Turning Self Criticism Into a Creative Asset* (New York: HarperOne, 1993), and Anna Katharina Schaffner, "Living with Your Inner Critic: 8 Helpful Worksheets and Activities," *Positive Psychology*, https://positivepsychology.com/inner-critic-worksheets.

4. "What's the most painful thing you've been told? (Strangers Answer)," YouTube, accessed February 8, 2022, https://www.youtube.com/watch? v=Dr10kEq-eu4&ab_channel=ThorayaMaronesy.

CHAPTER 4: CONNECTING WITH YOURSELF

1. An essay by Atul Gawande, the former United States surgeon general, can be found here: Atul Gawande, "On Washing Hands," *New England Journal of Medicine* 350 (March 25, 2004): 1283–86. https://doi.org/10.1056 /NEJMp048025. See also Carla Fried, "Hospital Hand-Washington: The Limits of Electronic Monitoring," *UCLA Anderson Review*, February 21, 2018, https://www.anderson.ucla.edu/faculty-and-research/anderson -review/hand-washing.

2. One page about the Three Pills can be found here: Tenzin Wangyal Rinpoche, "Remedy for Pain: Three 'Pills' of Inner Refuge," *Voice of Clear Light*, accessed December 15, 2021, http://www.voiceofclearlight.org/2012 /june/318-remedy-for-pain. For a five-minute video of Tenzin Wangyal describing the Three Pills see: Tenzin Wangyal Rinpoche, "The Three Pill Meditation Technique," *Study Buddhism*, accessed December 15, 2021, https://www.youtube.com/watch?v=Go7wT-2McdQ.

3. Compassion is the recognition of suffering in ourselves and others and the desire to try to what we can to relieve it. Self-compassion is defined by Kris-

tin Neff as "being open to and moved by one's own suffering, experiencing feelings of caring and kindness toward oneself, taking an understanding, non-judgmental attitude toward one's inadequacies and failures, and recognizing that one's experience is part of the common human experience." Kristin Neff, *Self-Compassion: The Proven Power of Being Kind to Yourself* (New York: William Morrow, 2015).

4. Kristin Neff, "The Space Between Self-Esteem and Self Compassion," *TEDx Talks*, February 6, 2013, https://www.youtube.com/watch?v=IvtZBUSplr4&ab_channel=TEDxTalks; Kristin Neff and Christopher Germer, *The Mindful Self Compassion Workbook: A Proven Way to Accept Yourself, Build Inner Strength, and Thrive* (New York: Guilford Press, 2018), 21–22.

5. Kristin Neff, "The Development and Validation of a Scale to Measure Self-Compassion," *Self and Identity* 2, no. 3 (2003): 223–50, https://doi.org/10.1080/15298860309027.

6. An extensive list of research studies on self-compassion can be found at https://self-compassion.org/the-research. More information on Neff, Gerner, and the program is available at https://self-compassion.org/the-program.

7. National Academy of Medicine, *Taking Action Against Clinician Burnout: A Systems Approach to Professional Well-Being* (Washington, DC: National Academies Press, 2019), https://doi.org/10.17226/25521.

8. Ciro Conversano et al., "Mindfulness, Compassion and Self-Compassion Among Health Care Professionals: What's New? A Systematic Review," *Frontiers in Psychology* 11, no. 5 (2020), https://doi.org/10.3389/fpsyg.2020.01683.

9. Kathi J. Kempter et al., "Do Mindfulness and Self-Compassion Predict Burnout in Pediatric Residents?" *Academic Medicine* 94, no. 6 (2019): 876–84, https://doi.org/10.1097/acm.0000000000002546.

10. Kristin D. Neff, Marissa C. Knox, Phoebe Long, and Krista Gregory, "Caring for Others without Losing Yourself: An Adaptation of the Mindful Self-Compassion Program for Healthcare Communities," *Journal of Clinical Psychology* 76, no. 9 (2020): 1543–62, https://doi.org/10.1002/jclp.23007.

11. Dorian Peters and Rafael Calvo, "Compassion vs. Empathy: Design for Resilience," *Interactions* 21, no. 5 (2014): 48–53, https://doi.org/10.1145/2647087.

12. Neff and Germer, *The Mindful Self Compassion Workbook*, 141–43.

13. Rinske A. Gotink et al., "Mindfulness and Mood Stimulate Each Other in an Upward Spiral: A Mindful Walking Intervention Using Experience Sam-

pling," *Mindfulness* 7, no. 5 (2016) 1114–22, https://doi.org/10.1007/s12671
-016-0550-8.

14. M. Teut et al., "Mindful Walking in Psychologically Distressed Individuals: A Randomized Controlled Trial," *Evidence-Based Complementary and
Alternative Medicine* 2013 (2013): 1–7, https://doi.org/10.1155/2013/489856.

15. Andrew Thurston, "Mindful Walking: a Tai Chi-Inspired Technique Could
Help People with Knee Osteoarthritis Walk More Without Further Damaging Their Joints," *The Brink*, January 15, 2019, http://www.bu.edu/arti
cles/2019/mindful-walking/.

16. Sabbi Lall, "Hearing through the Clatter," *MIT News*, September 9, 2019,
https://news.mit.edu/2019/hearing-through-clatter-auditory-processing
-0909.

17. Jan Chozen Bays, *How to Train a Wild Elephant and Other Adventures in
Mindfulness* (Boulder, CO: Shambhala Publications, 2011), 49–51.

18. Zahirul Islam's, Douglas Johnson's, and Pooya Jazayeri's replies to "Can you
auscultate properly through clothing?" Quora, July 7, 2017, https://www
.quora.com/Can-you-auscultate-properly-through-clothing?share=1.

In a 2017 online discussion about the question, "Can you auscultate
properly through clothing?" Dr. Pooya Jazayeri, a board-certified anesthesiologist, wrote:

> It's more accurate to auscultate with the stethoscope directly up against
> the skin. That doesn't mean it always needs to be done that way. A Fer-
> rari is faster than a Toyota. That doesn't mean you need a Ferrari to go to
> the grocery store, right? If it's a pulmonologist trying to tease out a faint
> expiratory wheeze or something then I would expect a very thorough
> auscultation of the chest. If I'm just checking to hear if breath sounds
> are present or not then listening through the clothing may be fine.
>
> If you ask an internist, or the doctor who taught me physical exam,
> then the clothing should always be removed. You want to inspect the
> entire patient so you don't miss a surgical scar or some other lesion. You
> also want to percuss and auscultate properly. In the real world, that's just
> not practical because we don't have an hour to examine every patient.

Dr. Douglas Johnson, a retired general surgeon wrote:

> It depends on how good you are at listening and how thoroughly you do
> it. To be frank, many physicians do this as a symbolic gesture to demon-

strate that they are doing their job. I suspect most modern-trained Western physicians can hardly recognize rales vs. rhonchi let alone explain the significance of the difference. I listen for rales at the bases and wheezes in the front to screen for CHF, pneumonia and COPD/asthma. I don't notice much difference between listening directly on the skin vs through the clothing.

Dr. Zahirul Islam, a pathologist, wrote:

Modern Stethoscopes are pretty darn good. In a Muslim country like Bangladesh we have to auscultate over thick layers of clothing on daily basis, because our ladies are pretty shy and they wouldn't let you (examine) them bare-chested. I am not implying that auscultation over clothing is as good as over bare skin but we are accustomed to it. And be sure our ears are pretty expert.

19. This study used a lung sound platform and showed that lung sounds were attenuated by 5–18 dB when two layers of cloth were placed between the stethoscope and the platform. This reduction was eliminated by firm pressure on the stethoscope. The authors warn that clothing can produce acoustic artifacts, and hinder accurate inspection and percussion. Steve Kraman, "Transmission of Lung Sounds Through Light Clothing," *Respiration* 75, no.1 (2008): 85–88, https://doi.org/10.1159/000098404.

20. Michael Craig Miller, "In Praise of Gratitude," *Harvard Health Publishing*, November 21, 2012, https://www.health.harvard.edu/blog/in-praise-of-gratitude-201211215561.

21. Roger Ulrich, "View Through a Window May Influence Recovery from Surgery" *Science* 224, no. 4647 (April 1984): 420–442. https://science.sciencemag.org/content/224/4647/420.

22. An extensive review of the research and literature on the benefits of nature on human health and well-being can be found at https://ellisonchair.tamu.edu/benefitsofplants/ and https://www.terrapinbrightgreen.com/reports/14-patterns/#footnote-001.

23. Biophilia is an innate connection to nature and living systems. The term was coined by biologist E. O. Wilson in this book: E. O. Wilson, *Biophilia* (Boston: Harvard University Press, 1984); ecotherapy, also known as nature therapy or green therapy, is the applied practice of the emergent field of ecopsychology, which was developed by Theodore Roszak. Ecotherapy

is based in the belief that people are part of the web of life and that our psyches are not isolated or separate from our environment. Ecopsychology is informed by systems theory. It asks people to explore their relationship with nature—an area not addressed in most types of psychotherapy. Some professionals exclusively teach and practice ecopsychology, while other mental health practitioners incorporate aspects of ecotherapy into their existing practices. See "Ecotherapy/Nature Therapy," GoodTherapy, https://www.goodtherapy.org/learn-about-therapy/types/econature-therapy; Richard Louv, "What is Nature-Deficit Disorder?" Children & Nature Network, October 2019, https://www.childrenandnature.org/resources/what-is-nature-deficit-disorder/.

24. Qing Li, *Forest Bathing: How Trees Can Help You Find Health and Happiness* (New York: Penguin Random House, 2018).

25. Tytti Pasanen, Liisa Tyrväinen, and Kalvei Korpela, "Perceived Health and Activity in Nature," *Applied Psychology: Health and Well-Being* 6, no. 3 (2014): 324–46, https://doi.org/10.1111/aphw.12031; University of Exeter, "Two Hours a Week Is Key Dose of Nature for Health and Wellbeing," *Science News*, June 13, 2019, https://www.sciencedaily.com/releases/2019/06/190613095227.htm.

26. Association of Nature and Forest Therapy Guides and Programs, https://www.natureandforesttherapy.earth/.

27. Wilson, *Biophilia*.

28. Paul Lecat et al., "Improving Patient Experience by Teaching Empathic Touch and Eye Gaze: A Randomized Controlled Trial of Medical Students," *Journal of Patient Experience* 7, no. 6 (2020): 1260–70, https://doi.org/10.1177/2374373520916323; Enid Montague et al., "Nonverbal Interpersonal Interactions in Clinical Encounters and Patient Perception of Empathy," *Journal for Participatory Medicine* 5:e33 9 (August 14, 2013), https://participatorymedicine.org/journal/evidence/research/2013/08/14/nonverbal-interpersonal-interactions-in-clinical-encounters-and-patient-perceptions-of-empathy/.

29. Dacher Keltner, "Hands on Research: The Science of Touch," Greater Good, Accessed November 28, 2021, https://greatergood.berkeley.edu/article/item/hands_on_research.

30. A review of the benefits of touch and massage therapy by Tiffany Field, director of the Touch Research Institute at the University of Miami School of Medicine. Tiffany M. Field, "Touch Therapy Effects on Development," *Inter-*

national Journal of Behavioral Development 22, no. 4 (December 1998): 779–97; Sheldon Cohen, Denise Janicki-Deverts, Ronald B. Turner, and William J. Doyle, "Does Hugging Provide Stress-Buffering Social Support? A Study of Susceptibility to Upper Respiratory Infection and Illness," *Psychological Science* 26, no.2 (2015): 135–47, https://doi.org/10.1177/0956797614559284.

31. James A. Coan, Hillary S. Schaefer, and Richard J. Davidson, "Lending a Hand: Social Regulation of the Neural Response to Threat," *Psychological Science* 17, no. 12 (2006): 1032–39, https://doi.org/10.1111/j.1467-9280.2006.01832.x.

32. Michael W. Kraus, Cassey Huang, and Dacher Keltner, "Tactile Communication, Cooperation, and Performance: An Ethological Study of the NBA," *Emotion* 10, no. 5 (October 2010): 745–49, https://doi.org/10.1037/a0019382.

33. Jan Chozen Bays, *Mindful Eating: A Guide to Rediscovering a Healthy and Joyful Relationship with Food* (Boulder, Colorado: Shambhala Publications, 2017).

34. Everything has a life story that is interesting, if we are curious. For the history of baking powder and how it is manufactured, see "Baking Powder," How Products Are Made, Accessed November 30, 2021, http://www.madehow.com/Volume-6/Baking-Powder.html.

35. A TEDMED Live talk by Dr. Madan Kataria, the founder of Laughter Yoga, accessed December 15, 2021, https://www.youtube.com/watch?v=5hf2umYCKr8. Without advertising, laughter yoga has spread to over twenty thousand free laughter groups in 110 countries; Heidi H. Beckman, Nathan Regier, and Judy Young, "Effect of Workplace Laughter Groups on Personal Efficacy Beliefs," *J Prim Prev* 28, no. 2 (March 2007):167–182, https//doi.org/10.1007/s10935-007-0082-z. A list of findings of recent research on Laughter Yoga can be found at American School of Laughter Yoga, "10 Academic Research on Laughter Yoga," accessed December 15, 2021, https://www.laughteryogaamerica.com/learn/research/academic-research-laughter-yoga-coming-4190.php.

36. The original Monty Python sketch: "Monty Python Ministry of Silly Walks," accessed November 30, 2021, https://www.youtube.com/watch?v=F3UGk9QhoIw.

37. Gomerblog.com is a funny, satirical website written by and for medical professionals.

38. Eino Partanen et al., "Fetal Brain Learns to Process Speech," *Proceedings of the National Academy of Sciences* 110, no. 37 (Sep. 2013): 15145–50, https://doi.org/10.1073/pnas.1302159110.

39. Jeonghee Kim et al., "The Tongue Enables Computer and Wheelchair Control for People with Spinal Cord Injury," *Science Translational Medicine* 5, no. 213 (2013), https://doi.org/10.1126/scitranslmed.3006296.

40. Caroline Bologna, "How to Stop Touching Your Face," HuffPost, March 2, 2020, https://www.huffpost.com/entry/how-to-stop-touching-your-face_l_5e59555ac5b6010221103ado?ncid=newsltushpmgnews.

41. Yen Lee Kwok, Angela Jan Gralton, and Mary-Louise McLaws, "Face Touching: A Frequent Habit That Has Implications for Hand Hygiene," *American Journal of Infection Control* 43, no. 2 (February 2015): 112–14, https://doi.org / 10.1016/j.ajic.2014.10.015.

42. Robert Emmons, "A Readable Review of Research Showing the Benefits of Clarifying Personal Goals or Strivings and Ultimate Concerns," in *The Psychology of Ultimate Concerns* (New York: Guilford Press, 1999), 103–104.

43. For relevant research and many stories of the vows of ordinary and famous people, see Jan Chozen Bays, *The Vow-Powered Life: A Simple Method for Living Life with Purpose* (Boston: Shambhala Publications, 2016).

44. Thanh Neville, M.D., "I'm an ICU Doctor and I Cannot Believe the Things Unvaccinated Patients Are Telling Me," HuffPost, August 1, 2021, https://www.huffpost.com/entry/icu-doctor-health-care-workers-unvaccinated-patients_n_6102ad2ae4b000b997df1f17; Eric Berger, "US Hospitals Outfitting Nurses with Panic Buttons amid Rise in Assaults," The Guardian, Guardian News and Media, September 30, 2021, https://www.theguardian.com/us-news/2021/sep/30/hospitals-nurses-panic-buttons-to-security.

CHAPTER 5: CONNECTING WITH YOUR PATIENTS

1. Stephan Duschek et al., "Dispositional Empathy Is Associated with Experimental Pain Reduction During Provision of Social Support by Romantic Partners," *Scandinavian Journal of Pain* 20 (August 2019): 205–209, https://doi.org 10.1515/sjpain-2019-0025.

2. I use the terms *empathy* and *compassion* here. For the current thinking about the difference between empathy fatigue and compassion fatigue, see the section on Mindful Self-Compassion.

3. Kathleen Gaines, "Nurses Ranked Most Trusted Profession Nineteen Years in a Row," Nurse.org, January 19, 2021, https://nurse.org/articles/nursing-ranked-most-honest-profession/.

4. Enid Montague et al., "Nonverbal Interpersonal Interactions in Clinical Encounters and Patient Perceptions of Empathy," *Journal for Participatory*

Medicine 5:e33 (August 14, 2013), https://participatorymedicine.org/journal
/evidence/research/2013/08/14/nonverbal-interpersonal-interactions-in
-clinical-encounters-and-patient-perceptions-of-empathy.

5. Montague et. al., "Nonverbal Interpersonal Interactions in Clinical Encounters and Patient Perceptions of Empathy."

6. Montague et. al., "Nonverbal Interpersonal Interactions in Clinical Encounters and Patient Perceptions of Empathy."

7. Ali Venosa, "Labia Surgery Is the Latest Trend Among Teenage Girls; Why So Many Are Asking for the Cosmetic Surgery," Medical Daily, April 27, 2016, https://www.medicaldaily.com/labiaplasty-cosmetic-surgery-teenage
-girls-383835.

8. *The World of Relaxation* by Jon Kabat-Zinn can be found at https://www
.mindfulnesscds.com/pages/hospital-dvd-cd.

9. John Zarb, Michelle Rickman, Steve Bongard, and David Powell, "Patient-Centered Approach to Dentistry: Essential. Inevitable. Achievable," OralHealth, November 12, 2019, https://www.oralhealthgroup.com/
features/patient-centred-approach-to-dentistry-essential-inevitable
-achievable.

10. See DonateContacts.com. Donate Contacts is an organization founded by teens. It focuses on ending the enormous waste of contact lenses worldwide and on providing underprivileged kids with access to free, quality contact lenses. They accept unused contact lens solution and contact lens cases. As of March 1, 2021, they have processed and donated over 2.3 million contact lenses, eleven thousand bottles of contact lens solution. and fifteen thousand contact lens cases.

11. Here's a link to a hobby information sheet for patients: www.shambhala
.com/mindfulmedresources. You can also find this sheet on p. 209.

12. Sarah Pressman et al., "Association of Enjoyable Leisure Activities with Psychological and Physical Well-Being," *Psychosomatic Medicine* 71, no. 7 (2010): 725–32, https://doi.org/10.1097/PSY.0b013e3181ad7978.

13. Xinyi Lisa Qian, Careen M. Yarnal, David M. Almeida, "Does Leisure Time as a Stress Coping Resource Increase Affective Complexity? Applying the Dynamic Model of Affect (DMA)." *Journal of Leisure Research* 45, no. 3 (2013): 393–414, https://doi.org/10.18666/jlr-2013-v45-i3-3157.

14. "How Personal Interests and Hobbies Influence Physicians at Work," Doximity, January 24, 2017, https://blog.finder.doximity.info/how-personal
-interests-and-hobbies-influence-physicians-at-work.

15. Jennifer Reiling, "The Hobbies of Physicians," *JAMA* 300, no. 9 (2008): 1008, https://doi.org/10.1001/jama.300.9.1088-a.

16. Amy Farouk, "How Physicians Spend Their Time Outside the Exam Room," *AMA Physician Health* (blog), December 26, 2014, https://www.ama-assn .org/practice-management/physician-health/how-physicians-spend -their-time-outside-exam-room.

17. John D Kelly IV, "Blog: Hobbies Are the Fun Way to Avoid Burnout," Healio, April 5, 2017, https://www.healio.com/news/orthopedics/20200408/blog -hobbies-are-the-fun-way-to-avoid-burnout. (A blog from an orthopedic surgeon who moonlights as a stand-up comedian.)

18. Kelly IV, "Blog: Hobbies Are the Fun Way to Avoid Burnout."

19. Are diagonal earlobe creases a sign of coronary artery disease? For a meta-analysis of the research see Aris P. Agouridis, Moses S. Elisaf, Devaki R. Nair, and Dimitri P. Mikhailidis, "Ear Lobe Crease: A Marker of Coronary Artery Disease?" *Archives of Medical Science* 11, no. 6 (2015): 1145–55, https://doi.org/10.5114/aoms.2015.56340. Conclusion: "After considering all the evidence, we cannot state with confidence that ELC (ear lobe crease) represents a marker of CAD (coronary artery disease). However, we suggest that patients with ELC may benefit from being monitored more closely for the potential presence of CAD."

20. John M. Kelley et al., "The Influence of the Patient-Clinician Relationship on Healthcare Outcomes: A Systematic Review and Meta-Analysis of Randomized Controlled Trials," *PLoS ONE* 9, no. 4 (2014), https://doi .org/10.1371/journal.pone.0094207.

21. WebMD, "What Eye Color and Shape Say About Your Health," November 3, 2021, https://www.webmd.com/eye-health/ss/slideshow-eye-color-health; Anna E. Barón et al., "Interactions between Ultraviolet Light and MC1R and OCA2 Variants Are Determinants of Childhood Nevus and Freckle Phenotypes," *Cancer Epidemiology Biomarkers & Prevention* 23, no. 12 (December 1, 2014): 2829–39, https://doi.org/10.1158/1055-9965.epi-14-0633.

22. Barón et al., "Interactions between Ultraviolet Light and MC1R and OCA2 Variants Are Determinants of Childhood Nevus and Freckle Phenotypes."

23. Jonathan F. Bassett and James M. Dabbs Jr., "Eye Color Predicts Alcohol Use in Two Archival Samples," *Personality and Individual Differences* 31, no. 4 (2001): 535–39, https://doi.org/10.1016/s0191-8869(00)00157-4.

24. Montague et al., "Nonverbal Interpersonal Interactions in Clinical Encounters and Patient Perceptions of Empathy."

25. Alicia Raeburn, "10 Places Where Eye-Contact Is Not Recommended (10 Places Where the Locals Are Friendly)," *The Travel* (blog), September 12, 2018, https://www.thetravel.com/10-places-where-eye-contact-is-not -recommended-10-places-where-the-locals-are-friendly.

26. Rustin Moore, "The Power of a Pet | Rustin Moore – Youtube," The Power of a Pet, TEDxOhioStateUniversity, April 6, 2016, https://www.youtube.com /watch?v=-t4m6moobMY. A TEDx Talk with research backup by a dean of veterinary studies at Ohio State University on the importance of healthcare workers asking about or prescribing time with pets; National Institutes of Health, "The Power of Pets," U.S. Department of Health and Human Services, April 6, 2020, https://newsinhealth.nih.gov/2018/02/power-pets; "How to Stay Healthy around Pets," Centers for Disease Control and Prevention, September 15, 2021, https://www.cdc.gov/healthypets/keeping -pets-and-people-healthy/how.html.

27. Tove Fall et al., "Early Exposure to Dogs and Farm Animals and the Risk of Childhood Asthma," *JAMA Pediatr*ics 169, no. 11 (November 2015): e153219, https://doi.org/10.1001:jamapediatrics.2015.3219; NIH/National Institute of Allergy and Infectious Diseases, "Exposure to pet and pest allergens during infancy linked to reduced asthma risk," ScienceDaily, September 19, 2017, www.sciencedaily.com/releases/2017/09/170919102555.htm.

28. This site contains not only a lot of information about pet ownership but also other interesting information as well. Celia Miller, "Pet Ownership Statistics," September 24. 2021, https://spots.com/pet-ownership-statistics. Acessed December 2, 2021.

29. Alfonso Sollami et al., "Pet Therapy: An Effective Strategy to Care for the Elderly? An Experimental Study in a Nursing Home," Acta Biomed for Health Professions 88, no. 1-S (2017): 25–31, https://doi.org/10.23750/abm .v88i1-S.6281.

30. Nancy E. Edwards, Alan M. Beck, and Eunjung Lim, "Influence of Aquariums on Resident Behavior and Staff Satisfaction in Dementia Units," *Western Journal of Nursing Research* 36, no. 10 (March 17, 2014): 1309–22, https://doi.org/10.1177/0193945914526647.

31. Helen Louise Brooks et al., "The Power of Support from Companion Animals for People Living with Mental Health Problems: A Systematic Review and Narrative Synthesis of the Evidence," *BMC Psychiatry* 18, no. 1 (February 5, 2018), https://doi.org/10.1186/s12888-018-1613-2.

32. "Resources Available Regarding the Benefits of Plants, Gardens, and

Improved Landscapes," Ellison Chair in International Floriculture, May 20, 2021, https://ellisonchair.tamu.edu/benefitsofplants. This is a four-volume extensive review of research on the benefits of plants.

33. Judith Rodin and Ellen J. Langer, "Long-Term Effects of a Control-Relevant Intervention with the Institutionalized Aged," *Journal of Personality and Social Psychology* 35, no. 12 (January 1977): 897–902, https://doi.org /10.1037/0022-3514.35.12.897; Charles R. Hall and Madeline W. Dickson, "Economic, Environmental, and Health/Well-Being Benefits Associated with Green Industry Products and Services: A Review," *Journal of Environmental Horticulture* 29, no. 2 (June 1, 2011): 96–103, https://doi.org /10.24266/0738-2898-29.2.96.

34. Seong-Hyun Park and Richard H Mattson, "Plants in Post-Op Rooms: Ornamental Indoor Plants in Hospital Rooms Enhanced Health Outcomes of Patients Recovering from Surgery," *Journal of Alternative and Complementary Medicine* 15, no. 9 (September 2009): 975–80, https://doi: 10.1089 /acm.2009.0075.

35. Richard Mottershead and Marjorie Ghisoni, "Horticultural Therapy, Nutrition and Post-Traumatic Stress Disorder in Post-Military Veterans: Developing Non-Pharmaceutical Interventions to Complement Existing Therapeutic Approaches," *F1000Research* 10 (September 3, 2021): 885, https://doi.org /10.12688/f1000research.70643.1; Bo-Young Kim, Sin-Ae Park, Jong-Eun Song, and Ki-Cheol Son, "Horticultural Therapy Program for the Improvement of Attention and Sociality in Children with Intellectual Disabilities," *HortTechnology* 22, no. 3 (June 2012): 320–24, https://doi.org/10.21273/hort tech.22.3.320.

36. Neha Sharma, "Why Doctors Should Provide Active Listening," *KevinMD* (blog), December 27, 2017, https://www.kevinmd.com/blog/2017/12/doctors -practice-active-listening.html. KevinMD is a MedpageToday platform with articulate, thoughtful blogs (like this one), written by doctors, nurses, and medical students.

37. "Impact of Communication in Healthcare," Institute for Healthcare Communication, July 2011, https://healthcarecomm.org/about-us/impact-of -communication-in-healthcare.

38. There is research that shows that a careful history provides the information needed to make the diagnosis 75–82 percent of the time. Michael C. Peterson et al., "Contributions of the History, Physical Examination, and Laboratory Investigation in Making Medical Diagnoses," *Obstetrical*

and Gynecological Survey 47, no. 10 (October 1992): 711–12, https://doi
.org/10.1097/00006254-199210000-0013.

39. Julian Treasure is a communication expert whose TED Talk on "How to
Speak So People Want to Listen" is the sixth most popular TED Talk. He
emphasizes listening as a learned and conscious skill. Julian Treasure.
"How to Speak so That People Want to Listen," TEDGlobal 2013, June
2013; Julian Treasure, "5 Ways to Listen Better," TEDGLobal 2011, July
2011.

40. Anjel Vahratian, Stephen J. Blumberg, Emily P. Terlizzi, and Jeannine S.
Schiller, "Symptoms of Anxiety or Depressive Disorder and Use of Mental
Health Care among Adults during the COVID-19 Pandemic - United States,
August 2020–February 2021," Centers for Disease Control and Prevention,
April 1, 2021, https://www.cdc.gov/mmwr/volumes/70/wr/mm7013e2
.htm?s_cid=mm7013e2_w.

41. Ayelet Meron Ruscio et al., "Cross-Sectional Comparison of the Epidemiology of DSM-5 Generalized Anxiety Disorder across the Globe," *JAMA
Psychiatry* 74, no. 5 (May 1, 2017): 465–75, https://doi.org/10.1001/jama
psychiatry.2017.0056.

42. Jayne Leonard and Timothy J. Legg, "Symptoms, Signs, and Side Effects
of Anxiety," Medical News Today, July 18, 2018, https://www.medicalnews
today.com/articles/322510; James A. Blumenthal and Patrick J. Smith,
"Risk factors: Anxiety and Risk of Cardiac Events," *Nat Rev Cardiol* 7, no.
11 (2010): 606–608, https//doi.org/10.1038/nrcardio.2010.139.

43. Darien Kadens, "Understanding and Managing Patient Fear in the Hospital Setting," https://www.slideshare.net/Innovations2Solutions/under
standing-and-managing-patient-fear-in-the-hospital-setting.

44. Tricia Miller and M. Robin Dimatteo, "Importance of Family/Social Support and Impact on Adherence to Diabetic Therapy." *Diabetes, Metabolic
Syndrome and Obesity, Targets and Therapy* 6 (November 5, 2013): 421–26.
https://doi.org/10.2147/DMSO.S36368.

45. Michelle McCabe, "Impact of Family Presence in the Healthcare Setting," Liberty University, 2014 (unpublished thesis for honors program),
https://digitalcommons.liberty.edu/cgi/viewcontent.cgi?article=1481&
context=honors.

46. McCabe, "Impact of Family Presence in the Healthcare Setting."

47. Juleen Radakowski et al., "Caregiver Integration During Discharge Planning for Older Adults to Reduce Resource Use: A Metaanalysis," *Journal of*

the American Geriatric Society 65, no. 8 (August 3, 2017): 1748–55, https://doi.org. 10.1111/jgs.14873.

48. Ahmed Elkhaldi, "The Impact of Family Support on Recovery of Depressed Patients in Gaza Governorates" (2013) (Unpublished master's thesis in Community Mental Health), https://library.iugaza.edu.ps/thesis/107608.pdf.

49. "Schwarz Rounds and Membership," The Schwartz Center, February 6, 2020, https://www.theschwartzcenter.org/programs/schwartz-rounds.

50. The *Nature* series on public television has many absorbing, educational, amusing, and relaxing documentaries for all ages. My favorite is this one about raccoons: "Raccoon Nation," *Nature*, season 30 episode 7, https://watch.opb.org/video/nature-raccoon-nation.

51. Isobel Heyman, Holan Liang, and Tammy Hedderly, "COVID-19 Related Increase in Childhood Tics And Tic-Like Attacks," *Archives of Disease in Childhood* 106, no.5 (March 6, 2021):420–21, https://doi.org/10.1136/archdischild-2021-321748.

52. Diane Atwood, "A Child with Autism, Count the Blessings," *Catching Health* (blog), https://dianeatwood.com/a-child-with-autism/.

53. "The Blessings of Asperger's: 40 Positive Characteristics of Asperger Syndrome," My ASD Child, https://www.myaspergerschild.com/2010/10/the-blessings-of-aspergers-40-positive.html.

54. Ruth King, *Mindful of Race: Transforming Racism from the Inside Out* (Louisville, CO: Sounds True, 2018).

CHAPTER 6: GUIDED MEDITATIONS

1. BodyWorlds.com has a variety of educational exhibits of plastinated bodies in many countries. There are several similar exhibits such as *Bodies: The Exhibition* and *Bodies Revealed*.

2. There is a novel by Ursula Le Guin called *The Lathe of Heaven*. It is set in Portland, Oregon, and includes the consequences of an attempt to end prejudice by giving everyone the same skin color. From Amazon: "A classic science fiction novel by one of the greatest writers of the genre, set in a future world where one man's dreams control the fate of humanity. In a future world racked by violence and environmental catastrophes, George Orr wakes up one day to discover that his dreams have the ability to alter reality. He seeks help from Dr. William Haber, a psychiatrist who immediately grasps the power George wields. Soon George must preserve reality

itself as Dr. Haber becomes adept at manipulating George's dreams for his own purposes. But as you'd expect from Le Guin, there's no shortage of more social questions raised here, from the nature of peace to the dangers of global warming, all done within a great narrative that twists and turns underneath you."

CHAPTER 7: RESCUE REMEDIES FOR TIMES OF ACUTE NEED

1. Three breathing exercises and techniques recommended by Dr. Weil with video demonstrations can be found at https://www.drweil.com/health -wellness/body-mind-spirit/stress-anxiety/breathing-three-exercises.

2. Jenna Fletcher, "How to Use 4-7-8 Breathing for Anxiety," *Medical News Today*, February 12, 2019, https://www.medicalnewstoday.com/articles /324417; Pratibha Pradip Pandekar and Poovishnu Devi Thangavelu, "Effect of 4-7-8 Breathing Technique on Anxiety and Depression in Moderate Chronic Obstructive Pulmonary Disease Patients," *International Journal of Health Sciences and Research* 9, no. 5 (2019): 209–17, https://www .academia.edu/43624599/Effect_of_4_7_8_Breathing_Technique_on_Anxi ety_and_Depression_in_Moderate_Chronic_Obstructive_Pulmonary_Dis ease_Patients.

3. James Carmody and Ruth A. Baer, "Relationships between Mindfulness Practice and Levels of Mindfulness, Medical and Psychological Symptoms, and Well-Being in a Mindfulness-Based Stress Reduction Program," *Journal of Behavioral Medicine* 31, no. 1 (2008): 23–33, https://doi.org/10.1007 /s10865-007-9130-7; Dana Schultchen et al., "Effects of an 8-Week Body Scan Intervention on Individually Perceived Psychological Stress and Related Steroid Hormones in Hair," *Mindfulness* 10 (2019): 2532–43, https:// doi.org/10.1007/s12671-019-01222-7; Heather L. Rusch et al., "The Effect of Mindfulness Meditation on Sleep Quality: A Systematic Review and Meta-Analysis of Randomized Controlled Trials," *Annals of the New York Academy of Sciences* 1445, no. 1 (June 2019): 5–16, https://doi.org 10.1111 /nyas.13996; Michael Ussher et al., "Immediate Effects of a Brief Mindfulness-Based Body Scan on Patients with Chronic Pain," *Journal of Behavioral Medicine* 37, no. 1 (February 2014):127–34, https://doi.org/10.1007/s10865 -012-9466-5.

4. "*Dona nobis pacem*" is Latin for "Grant us peace." These phrases, "*Nada te turbe, nada te espante*" (Let nothing disturb you, nothing frighten you") and "*Ubi caritas et amor, Deus ibi est*" ("Where there is charity and love,

God is there") are two songs from Taize, an ecumenical religious community in France. Their religious services center on lovely, simple chants sung in many different languages. Over 100,000 youth from all over the world make pilgrimages to Taize every year from all over the world. You can hear these chants here: https://www.youtube.com/watch?v=g01-BoDD7CI&ab_channel=MostarTaize; and here: https://www.youtube.com/watch?v=G2027qpvfUc&ab_channel=PawełSzczęsny.

5. Jan Chozen Bays, *Jizo Bodhisattva: Guardian of Children, Travelers and Other Voyagers* (Boston: Shambhala Publications, 2003).

6. Robert D. Brook et al., "Beyond Medications and Diet: Alternative Approaches to Lowering Blood Pressure: A Scientific Statement from the American Heart Association," *Hypertension* 61, no. 6 (June 2013): 1360–83, https//doi.org/10.1161/HYP.0b013e318293645f; Fred Travis et al., "Effect of Meditation on Psychological Distress and Brain Functioning: A Randomized Controlled Study," *Brain and Cognition* 125 (August 2018): 100–105, https://doi.org/10.1016/j.bandc.2018.03.011.

7. Brian Rees, Fred Travis, David Shapiro, and Ruth Chant, "Significant Reductions in Posttraumatic Stress Symptoms in Congolese Refugees Within Ten Days of Transcendental Meditation Practice," *Journal of Traumatic Stress* 27, no.1 (2014): 112–15, https://doi.org/10.1002/jts.21883; Seung Suk Kang et al., "Transcendental Meditation for Veterans with Post-Traumatic Stress Disorder," *Psychological Trauma: Theory, Research, Practice, and Policy* 10, no. 6 (2018): 675–80, https://doi.org/10.1037/tra0000346.

8. Gil Fronsdale, "The Buddha as a Parent," accessed December 15, 2021, https://www.insightmeditationcenter.org/books-articles/the-buddha-as-a-parent.

9. For inspiration, see the original Monty Python sketch about the government Ministry of Silly Walks at https://www.youtube.com/watch?v=F3UGk9QhoIw.

CHAPTER 8: SUGGESTIONS FOR MINDFUL MEDICINE GROUPS AND RETREATS

1. "Mindfulness Based Stress Reduction," https://mbsrtraining.com and "MBSR: Mindfulness-Based Stress Reduction," https://www.brown.edu/public-health/mindfulness/ideas/mbsr-mindfulness-based-stress-reduction.

2. David A. Schroeder, et al., "A Brief Mindfulness-Based Intervention for Primary Care Physicians: A Pilot Randomized Controlled Trial," *Ameri-*

can Journal of Lifestyle Medicine 12, no. 1 (February 4, 2016): 83–91, https://doi.org/10.1177/1559827616629121.

3. "Self-Compassion," Self-Compassion.org, accessed December 15, 2021, https://self-compassion.org/the-program; "Welcome to Mindful Practice in Medicine," University of Rochester Medical Center, accessed December 15, 2021, https://www.urmc.rochester.edu/family-medicine/mindful-practice.aspx; "About Us," Stanford Medicine, accessed December 15, 2021, https://wellmd.stanford.edu/about.html.

4. See chapter 8, note 3.

5. See chapter 8, note 3.

About the Author

Jan Chozen Bays, MD, is a pediatrician, Zen teacher, wife, mother, and grandmother. She has studied and practiced Zen since 1973 and is a board member and participant of Mindful Medicine, a nonprofit offering mindfulness groups and retreats to healthcare providers in the Portland, Oregon, area.

Dr. Bays worked for thirty years at Legacy Children's Hospital in Portland, Oregon, in outpatient pediatrics and as a specialist in child abuse cases. She received her Zen training under the revered Zen master Taizan Maezumi Roshi and then under Shodo Harada Roshi, abbot of Sogen-ji monastery in Japan. She is the coabbot of the Great Vow Zen Monastery in Clatskanie, Oregon, and helped found Heart of Wisdom Zen Temple in Portland, Oregon. She has published articles in *Tricycle* and *Buddhadarma*, and she is the author of the books *Jizo Bodhisattva*, *How to Train a Wild Elephant*, *Mindfulness on the Go*, *The Vow-Powered Life*, *Mindful Eating*, and *Mindful Eating on the Go*. In her spare time she likes to bake bread, grow flowers, and play in a marimba band.

For more information, visit www.zendust.org.